The Facultative Carnivore Diet

Understanding Why Protein and Fat Support Human Biology

First Edition: April 2026
ISBN: 978-1-966035-09-1
Published by Elite Nutrition Research
EliteNutritionResearch.com

Medical Disclaimer:
This book is intended for informational purposes only and is not a substitute for professional medical advice, diagnosis, or treatment. The content provided is based on the author's research, knowledge, and personal opinions. Always seek the advice of your physician or other qualifi ed health provider with any questions you may have regarding a medical condition. Never disregard professional medical advice or delay in seeking it because of something you have read in this book.

The author and publisher are not responsible for any health issues or consequences resulting from the use or misuse of the information contained in this book. Individual results may vary, and the suggestions herein may not be suitable for everyone. Readers are encouraged to consult with healthcare professionals before making any changes to their diet, exercise, or lifestyle routines.

ELITE

NUTRITION RESEARCH

Elite Nutrition Research is a science-driven health and education company dedicated to understanding and optimizing human physiology at its most fundamental level. Our work is built on an architecture-first approach—examining how nutrients interact with cellular systems, membranes, energy production, and signaling pathways to shape overall health and performance. Rather than following trends, we focus on first principles, combining biochemical insight, formulation precision, and practical application to create both advanced nutritional products and in-depth educational systems.

Through our books, courses, and formulations, Elite Nutrition Research aims to give individuals direct access to the mechanisms that govern their biology empowering them to think clearly, act intentionally, and build lasting health from the inside out.

To explore our full system of products, courses, and research, visit:
www.elitenutritionresearch.com

Table of Contents

Introduction

Why Nutrition Feels Broken

The confusion begins before a meal ever reaches the mouth. The human body is a structured biological system built from proteins, lipids, minerals, water, and regulated electrical gradients, yet most nutrition advice is delivered as if food were a moral category, a voting bloc, or a branding exercise. One expert tells the public to fear saturated fat because blood lipids matter. Another tells the public to fear carbohydrates because insulin matters. A third warns about meat because long-term disease associations matter. A fourth tells people to eat more plants because fiber and phytochemicals matter. Each frame isolates one piece of physiology, lifts it out of the whole, and then speaks as if that one piece is the body. But the body does not run on isolated talking points. It has to digest, absorb, transport, store, oxidize, repair, signal, and clear. Any nutrition framework that locks onto one variable while ignoring the rest will eventually contradict another framework built on a different variable. The contradiction is not mysterious. It is built into the way the subject is being approached.

A large part of the problem is that modern nutrition advice usually begins too late in the sequence. It starts with outcomes instead of inputs, with weight change instead of tissue construction, with blood markers instead of digestion, with population slogans instead of human structure. The body does not encounter a dietary ideology when food enters the gut. It encounters a physical substance that must be chewed, acidified, emulsified, cleaved by enzymes, moved across an absorptive membrane, routed through the liver, distributed through blood, incorporated into tissue, or cleared as waste. A food can look impressive on a label and still deliver poorly in the intestine. A diet can produce short-term weight loss and still underfeed structural needs. A study can track an association and still fail to show what actually happened between the food matrix, the digestive tract, the bloodstream, and the target tissue. When the public is handed conclusions without the biological sequence that produced them, nutrition starts to feel unstable because the middle of the story has been removed.

The public conversation is also distorted by the fact that different institutions are asking different questions. Basic physiology asks what the body requires to build and maintain itself. Clinical medicine often asks what pattern seems associated with disease endpoints. Public health asks what guidance can be scaled across populations. Food companies ask what can be sold repeatedly. Media asks what will compress into a headline. These are not the same question, so they do not produce the same answer. A researcher may study a narrow endpoint under controlled conditions. A journalist may convert that narrow result into a universal dietary warning. A manufacturer may then build a product around the headline and market it as a solution. By the time the information reaches the person standing in a grocery aisle, the original biological question is gone. What remains is a simplified instruction stripped of context, mechanism, and hierarchy. That is how the public ends up surrounded by foods engineered for profit, labels engineered for reassurance, and advice engineered for speed.

Another source of contradiction is that modern nutrition language frequently treats all calories, all proteins, all fats, and all carbohydrates as if they behave interchangeably once swallowed. They do not. Protein arrives as amino acid architecture. It has to be denatured by stomach acid, cleaved by proteases, absorbed, and then used to rebuild enzymes, muscle, transport proteins, immune molecules, and connective tissue. Fat arrives as hydrophobic energy and membrane material. It has to be emulsified by bile, hydrolyzed by lipase, packaged into transport particles, and delivered through lymph and blood. Carbohydrate arrives with very different kinetics. Refined carbohydrate can move quickly, raise blood glucose quickly, and force a strong insulin response that changes storage, appetite, and energy access within minutes. These are different physiological events. When advice reduces them to abstract numbers or treats them as equal units in a calorie ledger, the body disappears behind the arithmetic. People then sense that something is wrong, because their lived experience does not match the simplistic model they were given.

The result is a nutrition landscape that feels broken because it is speaking in fragments while the body is operating as a whole. People are told to eat for heart health, gut health, weight loss, blood sugar control, longevity, microbiome diversity, cholesterol reduction, or hormonal balance, often as if each were a separate project. But the organism has only one digestive tract, one liver, one bloodstream, one set of kidneys, one nervous system, and one pool of structural nutrients to work with. The same meal has to pass through all of it. The way out of the confusion is to return to first principles and rebuild the subject from the ground up. What is the body made of. What raw materials does it need repeatedly. What foods deliver those materials in forms digestion can actually liberate and absorb. What foods create friction, distortion, instability, or extra clearing burden. Nutrition begins to make sense again when it is brought back into contact with anatomy, chemistry, and metabolic sequence. That is where this book begins.

Why Modern Nutrition Advice Is Contradictory

The contradiction begins with a category error. Nutrition is usually discussed as if it were a debate about opinions, food groups, or moral choices, when in reality it is a question of biological construction and metabolic handling. The body is not asking whether a diet is progressive, traditional, clean, balanced, low-fat, low-carb, plant-based, or ancestral. It is asking what entered the digestive tract, what enzymes and acids had to be deployed against it, what crossed the intestinal membrane, what reached the blood intact, what the liver had to process, what tissues could actually use, and what had to be neutralized or cleared. Modern nutrition advice rarely starts there. It usually starts after the fact, with a slogan, a public health rule, a food label, a disease association, or a body-weight outcome. Once the argument begins downstream, contradiction is unavoidable, because different observers are measuring different pieces of the same event and then speaking as if their fragment is the whole.

One camp looks at blood glucose and sees the instability created by refined carbohydrate. Another looks at circulating lipoproteins and sees the transport problem created by disordered fat handling. Another looks at food questionnaires and large population datasets and sees statistical associations between broad dietary patterns and disease endpoints decades later. Another looks at body weight and appetite and sees the role of hyper-palatable processed food in driving excess intake. None of these observations is automatically false. The problem is that each one can be turned into an isolated nutritional doctrine. Carbohydrate becomes the villain because insulin matters. Saturated fat becomes the villain because lipid transport matters. Meat becomes the villain because epidemiology sees a pattern. Processed food becomes the villain because appetite regulation breaks under industrial food conditions. The body, meanwhile, has to manage all of it at once. It has to digest protein, emulsify fat, absorb minerals, regulate glucose, build membranes, synthesize hormones, and clear waste through the kidneys and liver. Advice becomes contradictory the moment one regulatory problem is mistaken for the entire structure of human nutrition.

The confusion is amplified by the fact that the institutions speaking about food are not asking the same biological question. A physiologist asks what raw materials the organism requires to maintain tissue, generate energy, and preserve structural order. A clinician may ask what dietary pattern improves a narrow lab marker in a patient already carrying metabolic damage. A public health body asks what message can be scaled across millions of people in a simplified form. A food company asks what can be manufactured cheaply, marketed cleanly, and sold repeatedly. A journalist asks what can be compressed into a headline sharp enough to travel. Those are radically different filters. By the time nutrition information reaches the public, it has often passed from a narrow study, to a simplified interpretation, to a media story, to a product claim, to a dietary identity. The biological event that actually matters, food entering a human system and being processed through real organs, is buried under translation layers. People feel the contradiction because they are being handed conclusions detached from mechanism.

Another reason the advice splinters is that foods are constantly discussed as if label content were the same as biological yield. It is not enough for a food to contain protein, calcium, iron, omega-3, antioxidants, or fiber on paper. Digestion has to liberate those compounds from the food matrix. They have to remain chemically available in the gut lumen, the interior space of the intestine where digestion and absorption occur. They have to avoid being trapped by inhibitors, avoid being degraded, cross the intestinal lining, survive first-pass handling by the liver when relevant, and reach tissues in a usable form. A plant food can test rich in minerals and still yield little if those minerals are bound by phytate or oxalate. A fortified processed food can carry a list of added vitamins and still behave like a blood sugar disruptor with weak satiety and poor structural value. A low-fat product can improve a marketing narrative while worsening hunger and pushing the eater toward repeated intake.

This is where contradiction becomes visible in real life. One authority is speaking about nutrient presence. Another is speaking about metabolic consequence. Those are not the same event.

The time scale also changes the conclusion. A diet can produce short-term weight loss because it suppresses appetite, reduces food choice, or creates a temporary energy deficit, yet still fail to supply the full structural and regulatory needs of the body over time. Another diet can improve a single biomarker in the near term while creating instability elsewhere. The body can tolerate a great deal in the short run. That does not mean the input is ideal. There is a difference between what produces a visible effect over twelve weeks and what supports digestion, tissue repair, hormonal stability, and energy production year after year. Modern nutrition advice often collapses these time scales into a single argument. Rapid outcome and long-term biological fit are treated as if they were interchangeable. They are not.

This is why nutrition feels like a hall of mirrors. Each framework captures a real piece of physiology, then overextends it into a total explanation. The body gets reduced to glucose handling, or cardiovascular risk, or microbiome diversity, or calorie balance, or weight loss adherence, depending on who is talking. What disappears is the architecture. Humans are built from amino acids, lipids, minerals, water, and regulated signaling systems. Food has to be judged by what it supplies to that structure, what it destabilizes, what it burdens, and what remains after digestion and clearance are complete. Once nutrition is brought back to that standard, much of the contradiction begins to thin out. The noise comes from fragments. Clarity begins when the whole sequence is put back together.

Why the Public Conversation Starts with Diet Labels Instead of Human Structure

The public conversation starts with diet labels because labels are cheap. Human structure is not. A label can be packaged, repeated, sold, defended, and turned into identity with almost no biological literacy required. Low-fat, plant-based, keto, Mediterranean, carnivore, clean eating, balanced diet. These terms move fast because they compress a complex physiological event into a social shorthand. They tell the listener what tribe the speaker belongs to, what foods are morally favored, and what broad outcome is being promised. Human structure does not compress that easily. If the conversation began where it should begin, with the stomach, the pancreas, the liver, the intestinal membrane, the amino acid pool, the cell membrane, the thyroid, the kidney, the mitochondrial energy system, the discussion would immediately become harder to market and harder to simplify. It is much easier to tell the public that a diet is heart healthy, anti-inflammatory, ancestral, or sustainable than to explain what happens when a mixed meal hits the gastric lumen, what insulin does to fuel partitioning, how bile acids emulsify fat, how amino acids are absorbed, or why a food that contains minerals on paper may deliver little after binding and digestive interference. Labels survive because they are socially efficient. Physiology does not flatter that kind of speed.

This is not an accident of language. It is the natural outcome of how modern nutrition is produced and distributed. Public health institutions need broad messages that can be delivered to millions of people in a few sentences. Journalists need headlines that can survive the scroll. Food companies need claims that can fit on a package. Influencers need a frame that can be turned into a personality and repeated across videos, books, and meal plans. None of these systems are rewarded for beginning with tissue architecture or digestive sequence. They are rewarded for clarity at the level of branding, not clarity at the level of mechanism. So the public gets categories instead of structures. People are told to eat more whole grains, less saturated fat, more plants, fewer processed foods, more fiber, fewer carbs, more protein, depending on which messaging layer they happen to encounter. Each message may contain a fragment of truth, but the fragment arrives detached from the biological system that would tell the listener when that advice applies, when it fails, and what tradeoffs it creates.

Diet labels also dominate because they give people a sense of order in a field that otherwise feels technically intimidating. Human structure requires attention to sequence. Food has to be broken down mechanically, denatured chemically, cleaved enzymatically, moved across membranes, sorted by the liver, distributed through blood, incorporated into tissue, or filtered and excreted. That is real complexity. A label removes the sequence and offers a shortcut. It says this diet is the answer. This food group is the problem. This macronutrient is the key. The public is then taught to think in outward patterns rather than inward events. Instead of asking what the body is made from, what it can actually digest, what it absorbs efficiently, what destabilizes appetite, or what creates organ burden, people ask whether a food is paleo, vegan, keto-friendly, anti-inflammatory, or clean. The label becomes the lens, and once that happens, structure disappears. The organism is replaced by a slogan.

Another reason the conversation starts with labels is that labels protect people from having to confront biological mismatch. If the discussion begins with human structure, then every food has to answer a harder question. What does this actually supply in usable form. What does digestion have to do to liberate it. What percentage is absorbed. What else comes with it. What does it block. What tissue does it burden. What downstream regulation does it distort. Those questions strip away a great deal of nutritional theater. A cereal fortified with vitamins looks less impressive when the conversation shifts to refined starch, blood glucose excursion, weak satiety, and the need for repeated feeding. A leafy plant that tests high in minerals looks different when the discussion reaches oxalate binding, lumen chemistry, and urinary excretion burden. A protein bar with a good label can collapse quickly once digestion, amino acid balance, emulsifiers, sweeteners, and appetite signaling are brought into view. Labels preserve appearances. Structure exposes yield.

The deeper problem is that labels encourage people to think of diets as belief systems instead of biological strategies. Once a person says I am low-carb, I am plant-based, I am Mediterranean, I am carnivore, the conversation begins organizing around membership rather than mechanism. Defending the label becomes easier than examining the physiology. But the body does not eat identities. It receives molecules. It has to decide, moment by moment, what to digest, what to absorb, what to oxidize for energy, what to store, what to transform, and what to clear. That work is physical, not ideological. The stomach does not care whether a meal belongs to a recognizable diet pattern. The small intestine does not absorb according to a cultural narrative. The liver does not detoxify by food philosophy. When nutrition is rebuilt from human structure instead of diet labels, the subject becomes more demanding, but it also becomes more honest. The conversation slows down, and that is exactly what it needs. Clarity begins when the label loses control and the biology comes back into view.

Why Calories, Trends, and Food Rules Do Not Explain What the Body Is Actually Doing

The body does not experience food as a number, a trend, or a commandment. It experiences food as material entering a living processing system. That material has to be chewed, acidified, denatured, emulsified, cleaved by enzymes, transported across membranes, sorted by the liver, circulated through blood, incorporated into tissue, oxidized for energy, stored, transformed, or excreted. A calorie does not describe that sequence. It is a heat unit, a measurement of how much energy a food releases when burned under controlled conditions. But the body is not a furnace and digestion is not combustion. Food in the body is not dropped into a flame. It is exposed to hydrochloric acid, bile acids, proteases, lipases, transport proteins, hormonal signals, and organ-level triage. Protein is dismantled into amino acids that may become muscle proteins, enzymes, immune molecules, or glucose if the body needs it. Fat is emulsified into microscopic droplets, hydrolyzed into fatty acids, packaged into transport particles, and either burned, stored, or built into membranes. Carbohydrate is reduced to sugars, absorbed quickly or slowly depending on structure, and handled through insulin-mediated partitioning that can favor immediate oxidation, glycogen storage, or fat production when supply exceeds local demand. None of that is captured by a simple energy number.

This is why calorie thinking repeatedly fails to explain the lived experience of eating. Two meals can contain the same measured energy and still produce completely different biological results. A meal built from steak and eggs arrives with dense protein, fat, cholesterol, fat-soluble nutrients, and a digestion pattern that slows gastric emptying, stimulates satiety hormones, and supplies structural material the body can directly use. A meal built from sweetened cereal and skim milk may produce a much faster glucose rise, a stronger insulin response relative to its structural value, weaker satiety, and a quicker return of hunger. On paper the numbers may look manageable. In tissue they are not the same event. One meal provides amino acids and lipids that can be built into the organism. The other pushes the body through rapid fuel handling with far less structural payoff. The body does not ask how many calories entered the mouth in the abstract. It asks what chemistry arrived, how fast it arrived, what hormones were triggered, what nutrients were actually liberated from the food matrix, and whether the incoming material solved a biological need or merely flooded the system with disposable energy.

Trends fail for the same reason. They usually begin with a visible outcome and then mistake that outcome for an explanation. A low-fat trend emerges because one slice of physiology appears important, often blood lipids or cardiovascular risk language. A low-carb trend emerges because another slice becomes dominant, often glucose control, insulin exposure, or obesity. A plant-based trend emerges because fiber, phytochemicals, or epidemiologic associations become the organizing frame. Each trend grabs a fragment of the organism, then tries to govern the whole body through that fragment. But the organism is not a one-variable machine. It has to maintain nitrogen balance, membrane integrity, bile flow, thyroid output, mitochondrial ATP production, mineral status, immune surveillance, renal clearance, and stable fuel access at the same time. A dietary trend may improve one visible parameter while quietly degrading another. A person can lose weight on a restrictive trend and still underconsume protein. A person can improve glucose control temporarily while failing to supply fat-soluble nutrients or support digestion. A person can follow a food ideology with perfect discipline and still feed the body poorly if the nutrients delivered are incomplete, poorly absorbed, or paired with compounds that interfere with extraction and use. Trends survive because they are socially powerful. Biology remains harder because it forces a full accounting.

Food rules create a similar illusion of control. Eat six times a day. Do not eat after seven. Never combine this with that. Always eat breakfast. Avoid red meat. Choose whole grains. Everything in moderation. These rules feel useful because they simplify decisions, but they often hover above the mechanism instead of entering it. A rule may accidentally help because it reduces processed food, lowers refined sugar exposure, increases protein, or creates longer gaps between insulin surges. But the rule itself is not the explanation. The explanation is always physical. If eating less often helps, the question is what happened to insulin signaling, appetite oscillation, and digestive burden. If a higher-protein breakfast helps, the question is what happened to gastric emptying, glucagon balance, peptide YY, and later hunger. If removing refined carbohydrates helps, the question is what happened to blood glucose excursion, energy access, and repeated storage signaling. Rules are often shadows cast by mechanisms. People are handed the shadow and never shown the structure creating it.

The deeper issue is that calories, trends, and food rules all encourage the same mistake. They teach people to manage food from the outside instead of understanding what the body is doing on the inside. They reduce nutrition to arithmetic, fashion, or obedience. But the body is running a sequence, not following a slogan. It is evaluating amino acid availability, the rate of glucose entry, the stability of membrane lipids, the adequacy of micronutrient cofactors, the burden placed on liver detoxification and kidney filtration, and the hormonal meaning of the meal that just arrived. It does not care whether a plate conforms to the latest trend. It cares whether digestion can liberate usable material, whether tissues can absorb and retain it, and whether the net result supports structure, energy, and metabolic order. Once that becomes the standard, most of the noise begins to fall away. Calories can estimate potential energy. Trends can describe cultural patterns. Rules can organize behavior. None of them tell you what the organism is actually doing. Only physiology can do that.

The Governing Premise of the Book: Start with Physiology, Then Judge Food by Biological Fit

This book begins from a simple correction. Nutrition has been taught backward. Most modern food arguments begin with categories, recommendations, fears, outcomes, or identities. They begin with plant-based, low-fat, Mediterranean, balanced diet, superfood, processed food, anti-inflammatory food, clean food. They begin with the label attached to the food and then try to reason inward toward the body. Physiology forces the sequence to run in the opposite direction. The body comes first. The digestive tract, the liver, the pancreas, the gallbladder, the intestinal membrane, the bloodstream, the mitochondria, the kidneys, the endocrine system. These are the structures that food has to pass through and answer to. A food is not good because it carries a good reputation. It is not bad because it has been culturally condemned. It is biologically appropriate or biologically costly according to what the human organism has to do with it after ingestion. That is the governing premise here. Start with the organism, then judge the food.

Judging food by biological fit means asking a harder question than modern nutrition usually asks. Not what does the food contain on paper, but what can the body actually extract from it. What must digestion do first. Does the stomach need strong acid to denature it. Does fat need bile to emulsify it. Are the proteins complete and absorbable. Are the minerals chemically available in the gut lumen, the interior space of the intestine where digestion and absorption occur, or are they bound by other compounds before they ever reach the membrane. Does the food deliver amino acids the body can build with, fats the body can oxidize and incorporate into membranes, vitamins and minerals in usable forms, or does it arrive with structural barriers, irritants, inhibitors, and disposal work. Food enters the mouth as matter from the outside world. It becomes nourishment only if the body can break it down, absorb it, transport it, retain it, and use it without creating more burden than value.

This is why physiology has to come first. The body is not nourished by ingredient lists, marketing narratives, or moral language. It is nourished by molecules that survive the digestive event and reach tissues in useful form. A food can test rich in nutrients and still feed the body poorly if those nutrients remain trapped in the matrix, bound in insoluble complexes, lost in poor absorption, or offset by compounds that increase irritation and excretion burden. A food can look light, clean, and modern and still destabilize appetite, blood glucose, and energy access. Another food can be culturally treated as heavy or primitive while delivering dense protein, highly bioavailable minerals, stable fuel, and strong satiety with relatively little digestive friction. The body does not respond to image. It responds to exposure, extraction, signaling, and yield.

Biological fit also means that the same food must be judged across the full sequence, not just at one stage. What enters the gut is only the beginning. The intestine has to absorb it. The liver has to process it. The blood has to carry it. Cells have to use it. The kidneys may have to clear part of it. A food that looks acceptable at the level of calories may perform badly at the level of hormonal stability. A food that seems rich in micronutrients may create a poor net result once binding, inhibition, and renal burden are included. A food that gives a rapid subjective lift may still be a bad trade if it drives repeated insulin spikes, unstable appetite, and weak tissue support. This book will keep returning to that standard because it is the only standard that makes the contradictions of modern nutrition begin to resolve. The real question is never whether a food sounds healthy. The real question is what the body is left with after the full biological event is over.

From that premise, the rest of the argument follows naturally. If humans are built from amino acids, lipids, minerals, water, and regulated signaling systems, then foods should be ranked according to how directly and efficiently they supply those materials. If digestion is a real physical bottleneck, then digestibility and bioavailability matter more than label claims. If tissues require stable inputs to maintain energy production, membrane integrity, hormone synthesis, and repair, then foods that reliably provide those inputs deserve a different status from foods that are merely tolerated. This is the frame of the book. Physiology first. Biological fit second. Everything else, dietary tribe, cultural prestige, food mythology, trend language, comes after that or not at all.

What the Facultative Carnivore Framework Means and Why It Changes How the Reader Sees Food

The term facultative carnivore describes a pattern of biological preference with retained flexibility. Facultative means capable of functioning under more than one condition without implying that all conditions are equally good. In physiology, flexibility is not the same thing as design priority. The human body can metabolize carbohydrates, tolerate a range of plant foods, and survive across very different food environments. That much is obvious. But survival capacity does not settle the deeper nutritional question. The real issue is which foods most directly supply the materials the body is built from, which foods digestion can process with the least distortion, and which foods deliver the highest usable yield once absorption, transport, and tissue use are taken into account. The facultative carnivore framework argues that animal foods occupy the center of that picture because they provide dense protein, complete amino acid profiles, highly usable fats, and a broad range of vitamins and minerals in forms that align closely with human digestive and metabolic systems. Plant foods may still be eaten, but they move out of the foundation and into the category of optional inputs whose value depends on preparation, dose, tolerance, and tradeoff.

That shift changes the way food is judged. In the standard public frame, foods are usually organized by cultural categories. Fruits and vegetables are treated as automatically healthful. Whole grains are treated as staple-worthy. Meat is often treated as risky or secondary, something that must be defended or limited. The facultative carnivore frame does not begin with those reputations. It begins with digestive workload and biological yield. What happens when the food reaches the stomach. Does it require strong acid and proteolysis, the enzymatic cutting of proteins into absorbable fragments, in order to release amino acids the body can immediately use. Does it contain fat that bile can emulsify and the intestine can absorb into lymphatic transport particles. Or does it arrive with fiber-bound structures, mineral binders, enzyme inhibitors, fermentable substrates, and defense chemicals that the body must work around before it can access a smaller pool of useful nutrition. Under this framework, the question is no longer whether a food belongs to a protected category. The question is what it costs the organism to get nourishment out of it, and what the organism is actually left with after that work is complete.

It also changes how the reader thinks about plant foods. In the usual nutrition conversation, plant foods are treated as mandatory anchors of the diet and animal foods are treated as optional additions. The facultative carnivore framework reverses the hierarchy. Animal foods become the structural base because they provide the most direct route to amino acids, bioavailable iron, zinc, vitamin B12, cholesterol for steroid hormone synthesis, and fats that can be oxidized for energy or incorporated into membranes with relatively little digestive friction. Plant foods stop being assumed necessities and start being evaluated for compatibility. Some may be tolerated well in modest amounts. Some may provide useful carbohydrates or culinary variety. Others may create digestive irritation, unstable appetite, mineral interference, oxalate burden, glycemic instability, or simple displacement of better foods. This is not a moral demotion of plants. It is a physiological reclassification. Once the reader sees that a food can be edible without being foundational, the entire map of nutrition changes.

The framework also breaks the spell of the omnivore label. Omnivore only tells you that humans can consume both plant and animal matter. It says almost nothing about hierarchy, efficiency, or preferred fuel structure. The facultative carnivore model is more precise because it distinguishes between tolerance and fit. The body can use many foods in the way a system can endure many conditions. That does not mean all foods serve the structure equally well. The human digestive tract has a highly acidic stomach that denatures protein aggressively, a small intestine specialized for absorbing amino acids and fats, bile physiology built to manage lipid digestion, and metabolic pathways that can maintain blood glucose even when carbohydrate intake is low through gluconeogenesis, the endogenous production of glucose from non-carbohydrate substrates. That arrangement does not describe a body dependent on plant bulk as a first principle. It describes a body that can adapt broadly while still showing a strong nutritional advantage when fed dense animal-derived material.

Once the reader understands that, food stops looking like a debate between dietary identities and starts looking like a hierarchy of biological fit. The meal is no longer judged by whether it sounds balanced, clean, heart healthy, or culturally approved. It is judged by whether it feeds the organism cleanly, whether it stabilizes energy, whether it supplies structural nutrients in usable forms, and whether it minimizes unnecessary digestive and excretory burden. That is why this framework matters. It does not merely add another label to the crowded nutrition landscape. It removes the reader from label-thinking altogether and returns the subject to anatomy, digestion, and tissue economy. Food begins to look less like ideology and more like input. Once that happens, many things that used to seem confusing become much easier to see.

Part I

Leaving the Modern Nutrition Framework

Chapter 1

Why Nutrition Advice Often Conflicts

The public steps into nutrition through a field of competing authorities, each speaking from a different layer of the problem and each sounding complete from inside its own frame. The endocrinologist sees insulin, glucose handling, adipose storage, and metabolic syndrome. The cardiologist sees lipoproteins, vascular injury, inflammatory signaling, and long-term cardiovascular risk. The gastroenterologist sees reflux, malabsorption, bowel irritation, microbial imbalance, and altered transit. The sports nutrition specialist sees glycogen turnover, protein synthesis, recovery, and training output. The epidemiologist sees population-level dietary patterns and disease associations spread across years or decades. None of these views is invented. Each is observing something real. The confusion begins when a specialized window starts speaking as if it were the whole building. A body is not a blood sugar chart, a lipid panel, a colon, or a body-composition scan. It is an integrated organism that has to digest, absorb, transport, store, oxidize, repair, defend, and clear all at once. Advice starts to collide when narrow professional vision is mistaken for total nutritional truth.

This is why one expert can tell the public to restrict saturated fat because altered lipoprotein traffic matters, while another tells the public to restrict refined carbohydrate because insulin exposure and unstable glucose flux matter, while another pushes plant diversity because fermentation substrates and certain phytochemicals matter, while another prioritizes protein because lean tissue, satiety, and repair matter. All of them can point to real physiology. The problem is not that every expert is hallucinating. The problem is that each expert is often selecting the part of physiology most visible inside his own domain, then building dietary conclusions outward from that fragment. The fragment may be accurate. The hierarchy may still be wrong. A person can improve one biomarker while worsening appetite control. A diet can reduce one disease risk factor while degrading digestive comfort or structural nutrition. A food can perform well in one organ system and poorly in another. If the reader is never shown the full biological sequence from ingestion to tissue consequence, the advice lands as contradiction because the organism itself has been broken into disconnected specialties.

The public is then asked to make sense of food in a language built from these collisions. Fat is dangerous. Fat is essential. Meat is nutrient dense. Meat is inflammatory. Whole grains are foundational. Grains are metabolic stressors. Fruit is protective. Fruit is sugar delivery. Fiber is necessary. Fiber is irritating in the wrong gut. Calories matter most. Hormones matter most. The average person hears this as evidence that nutrition science is unserious or that experts are simply choosing teams. What is actually happening is more mechanical. Different expert systems are measuring different endpoints, on different time scales, in different populations, under different assumptions about what the body most needs protected. A physician dealing with advanced diabetes sees one pattern. A researcher studying frailty and muscle loss in aging sees another. A clinician treating inflammatory bowel symptoms sees another. A food manufacturer funding favorable framing sees something else again. These are not interchangeable vantage points. Once they are flattened into public nutrition messaging, they sound like open contradiction because the scaffolding underneath them has been removed.

Another source of confusion is that expert systems often disagree not only because they prioritize different organs, but because they start from different definitions of success. Is success lower body weight, lower fasting glucose, lower apolipoprotein B, better bowel regularity, fewer cravings, improved strength, lower medication burden, improved thyroid output, better iron status, or reduced kidney stone risk. The answer changes the advice. A food that looks helpful through one metric can become costly when the frame widens. A low-fat pattern may reduce one exposure while increasing hunger and weakening fat-soluble nutrient delivery. A high-fiber pattern may improve stool bulk while worsening bloating, mineral access, or bowel irritation in a compromised gut. A glucose-stabilizing pattern may work well for appetite and energy yet still require further refinement if protein intake, micronutrient density, or digestive tolerance are poor. Expert systems produce public confusion because the body is one structure but the culture of expertise is divided into compartments, each with its own favored endpoint and its own preferred explanation.

The way out is not to pick the loudest expert or the most fashionable specialty. It is to move beneath the specialties and return to the common substrate they are all trying, imperfectly, to describe. Food enters the mouth as external matter. It is mechanically broken down, chemically processed, absorbed through intestinal tissue, routed through blood, sorted by the liver, distributed to cells, incorporated into structure or burned for energy, and whatever remains must be stored, neutralized, or excreted. That sequence happens whether the meal is praised by a cardiologist, condemned by an influencer, or hidden inside a government guideline. Once the reader begins with that physical sequence, much of the conflict becomes easier to interpret. Experts are often seeing real pieces of reality. Public confusion begins when no one rebuilds the organism those pieces belong to.

he Difference Between Short-Term Diet Outcomes and Long-Term Biological Compatibility

Short-term diet outcomes are easy to see because they sit close to the surface. Body weight drops. Appetite falls for a few weeks. Water leaves the tissues. Blood glucose improves. A person feels lighter, less bloated, more in control, or more compliant because the food rules are clear and the novelty is still doing part of the work. None of that is meaningless, but none of it settles the deeper question of whether the diet actually fits the organism over time. A body can produce a quick visible response to many kinds of pressure. It can burn stored glycogen, reduce gut bulk, lower insulin exposure, suppress appetite under novelty, or tolerate a temporary narrowing of food choice. That is not the same thing as saying the diet is supplying the full set of materials needed for ongoing repair, hormone production, membrane maintenance, mineral balance, digestive stability, and durable energy production. The short run reveals adaptation. The long run reveals compatibility.

Biological compatibility is a harder standard because it forces the food pattern to answer to real tissue maintenance month after month, year after year. The question is not whether a person can lose weight quickly while following a system. The question is whether the digestive tract can keep extracting high-quality protein, usable fats, fat-soluble vitamins, bioavailable minerals, and adequate energy without accumulating hidden costs. Can lean mass be maintained. Can the body keep replacing enzymes, transport proteins, immune proteins, connective tissue, intestinal cells, and steroid hormones without robbing from its own reserves. Can the liver process the incoming chemistry without being buried under low-value food volume, unstable glucose traffic, or excessive detoxification work. Can the appetite system remain calm without constant discipline and psychological management. A diet may produce a dramatic early result while quietly underfeeding structural needs, weakening satiety, narrowing micronutrient coverage, or increasing dependence on willpower. The body can conceal those costs for a while. It cannot conceal them forever.

This is why so many diets look better at twelve weeks than they do at two years. In the beginning, almost any system that removes processed food, reduces random snacking, lowers refined carbohydrate exposure, or increases protein can create visible improvement. The body responds quickly when a major source of metabolic chaos is reduced. But long-term biological fit demands more than the removal of obvious damage. It demands sustained delivery of what the organism is built from. A person can lose weight on a low-fat diet and still struggle with satiety, fat-soluble nutrient handling, and hormone balance. A person can lose weight on a plant-heavy pattern and still deal with digestive friction, incomplete protein coverage, poor mineral yield, or rising dependency on fortification and supplementation. A person can stabilize blood sugar on a restrictive plan and still fail if the food pattern remains socially brittle, nutritionally thin, or structurally incomplete. Early success often reflects that a pressure was removed. Long-term success reflects that the right materials were supplied and the body could keep running on them without strain.

The difference matters because modern nutrition constantly confuses visible response with deep fit. It treats rapid movement as proof. But the organism is not asking whether a diet produced an impressive graph in the first quarter. It is asking whether the incoming food supports the continuous work of being alive. Cells still need membranes. Muscle still needs amino acids. Bile still needs to flow. Mitochondria still need usable fuel. Kidneys still need a manageable excretory load. Appetite still needs honest satiety signals instead of repeated manipulation. Long-term biological compatibility is therefore the higher test. It asks what remains after the excitement is over, after the water shift is gone, after the novelty fades, after the initial restriction stops carrying the system.

What remains is the real diet. What remains is the food pattern the body has to live inside.

How Nutrition Became an Ideological Fight Instead of a Physiological Question

Nutrition became ideological the moment the body was pushed out of the center of the discussion and replaced by symbols. Once that happened, food stopped being judged primarily by digestion, absorption, tissue use, and metabolic consequence, and started being judged by what it signaled socially. Meat came to represent one set of moral and political meanings. Plant foods came to represent another. Fat, sugar, grains, dairy, fasting, supplements, and even meal timing were gradually absorbed into larger identity systems. People no longer argued first about what the stomach has to do with a food, what the intestine can extract from it, what the liver must process after absorption, or what the cell can actually do with the incoming material. They argued about purity, restraint, sustainability, modernity, tradition, compassion, discipline, optimization, and belonging. Once food becomes symbolic, physiology loses authority. The digestive tract does not disappear in reality, but it disappears in the public mind. The question shifts from what nourishes the organism to what the eater wants to express by choosing it.

This shift was made easier by the structure of modern public discourse. Physiology is slow, layered, and technical. It requires the reader to follow a sequence from food structure to digestive event to hormonal response to tissue effect. Ideology is faster. It can compress an entire dietary worldview into a slogan, a label, or a prohibition. Eat clean. Cut carbs. Plants are medicine. Meat is toxic. Fat is dangerous. Seed oils are poison. The public can organize itself around those phrases immediately because they do not require a full mechanism. They require allegiance. And allegiance is emotionally efficient. A person can adopt a dietary identity long before he understands gastric acid, bile release, insulin signaling, amino acid sufficiency, mitochondrial fuel handling, or mineral bioavailability. That is how nutrition stopped being a question about what the body is made of and became a question about which side someone is on. The diet became a flag.

Institutions accelerated the change because ideology travels better than physiology through modern systems. Media needs conflict, not digestive chemistry. Food companies need narratives that make products feel virtuous or safe, not explanations of what refined starch does to blood glucose kinetics or what phytic acid does to mineral binding in the gut lumen. Public health messaging needs simplification that can survive mass distribution, which means it often speaks in food categories and moral shorthand rather than tissue-level detail. Advocacy groups naturally defend the dietary pattern that supports their ethical or cultural commitments. Even individuals do it in smaller form. Once a person has reorganized his routines, social world, and self-image around a dietary pattern, changing his nutritional view no longer feels like updating a model. It feels like betraying a camp. At that point, contradictory evidence is no longer weighed primarily for biological accuracy. It is screened for threat. The argument becomes tribal before it becomes anatomical.

The cost of this ideological turn is that foods stop being judged by net biological yield. A plant food may be defended because it belongs to the right moral category even if it binds minerals, irritates a damaged gut, or delivers weak structural nutrition relative to its reputation. An animal food may be attacked because it belongs to the wrong symbolic category even if it supplies dense protein, bioavailable iron, vitamin B12, cholesterol for steroid synthesis, and fats the body can use directly. A processed product may be protected because it has the right label language even when it destabilizes appetite and floods the system with rapidly absorbable energy. Ideology does this by flattening the sequence. It removes the stomach, the pancreas, the liver, the membrane, the mitochondrion, and the kidney from the conversation, then replaces them with moral abstractions. But the body does not live in abstractions. It lives in chemistry, tissue turnover, and continuous metabolic triage. The way back is to drag the argument out of identity and return it to the organism. Food is not a political philosophy. It is incoming matter that either fits human physiology cleanly or forces the body to pay for the mismatch.

Why the Body Does Not Care About Diet Identities

The body does not recognize keto, vegan, paleo, Mediterranean, carnivore, clean eating, or balanced diet as biological categories. It recognizes molecules, mechanical events, and regulatory signals. A meal enters the mouth as external matter. It is chewed into smaller particles, mixed with saliva, exposed to stomach acid, denatured, emulsified, cleaved by enzymes, moved through the intestinal lumen, absorbed across epithelial membranes, routed through the portal vein to the liver, sorted, stored, oxidized, incorporated into tissue, or cleared as waste. That entire sequence unfolds without reference to ideology. The stomach does not lower its pH because a food belongs to a respected dietary tribe. The gallbladder does not release bile because a meal carries a good cultural reputation. The intestine does not absorb iron, amino acids, glucose, or fatty acids according to the name of the diet printed over the plate. The organism is dealing with chemistry and structure, not identity.

Diet identities matter socially because they simplify complexity. They tell people what foods belong, what foods are excluded, and what kind of person the eater is trying to be. But social shorthand is not the same thing as physiological truth. A food can belong to a highly praised dietary pattern and still perform poorly inside a human body. A plant-heavy pattern can look disciplined and virtuous while delivering incomplete protein, lower mineral availability, more digestive interference, and more conversion burden. A low-fat pattern can look medically respectable while weakening satiety, reducing fat-soluble nutrient absorption, and pushing the eater toward repeated carbohydrate exposure. A high-carb athletic pattern can improve training output in one context and destabilize appetite or glycemic control in another. The body does not reward consistency to a food ideology. It rewards compatibility between incoming material and the systems responsible for digestion, energy production, structural repair, and regulation.

This is why diet identity can become a trap. Once a person begins to think of himself as belonging to a dietary camp, food stops being judged by net biological yield and starts being judged by whether it fits the story. Contradictory bodily signals are then reinterpreted rather than examined. Persistent hunger gets explained away as poor discipline. Bloating becomes an adjustment phase. Falling energy becomes detox, healing crisis, adaptation, or the cost of doing the right thing. Weak recovery becomes something to push through. Instead of asking whether the body is actually receiving usable amino acids, stable fuel, absorbable minerals, adequate fat-soluble nutrients, and calm digestive signaling, the person asks whether he is following the rules faithfully enough. Identity protects the framework even while the organism is paying for it.

The body is indifferent to that loyalty because it has a different accounting system. It asks whether essential amino acids arrived in sufficient quantity and balance to support protein synthesis. It asks whether fats were delivered in forms that can be oxidized, stored, or incorporated into membranes. It asks whether blood glucose rose in a manageable range or whether insulin had to work repeatedly to contain a fast fuel load. It asks whether minerals remained soluble in the gut or were trapped by phytate, oxalate, or other binding compounds before absorption could occur. It asks whether the liver received a manageable stream of nutrients and toxins or whether it was handed constant disposal work. It asks whether the kidneys are clearing routine waste or also bearing the burden of compounds the body cannot meaningfully use. This is the level where food is actually judged. Biological fit lives here. Dietary identity does not.

Once this is understood, the reader can stop asking whether a food belongs to the correct philosophy and begin asking what the food does inside a human system. That question is slower, less tribal, and far more useful. It pulls attention away from branding and back toward anatomy. It shifts the standard from symbolic compliance to physiological consequence. The body does not care what the eater calls himself. It cares what crossed the membrane, what reached the cells, what supported structure, what destabilized regulation, and what had to be cleared after the meal was over. That is the only nutrition language the organism speaks.

Chapter 2

Diet Culture vs Biological Understanding

Diet culture emerged when food was pulled away from physiology and attached to appearance, control, and public virtue. For most of human history, eating was constrained by season, labor, local ecology, animal access, storage limits, and the simple need to remain physically functional. Food was a supply problem before it became an identity project. The body had to be fed well enough to maintain strength, fertility, repair, and endurance. That does not mean historical diets were perfect. It means the central question was still biological. What can be eaten. What sustains work. What preserves life through winter, illness, pregnancy, injury, and scarcity. Diet culture changed the frame. It made food less about structural sufficiency and more about body management under modern visual pressure. Once that happened, nutrition stopped being organized primarily around what tissues require and started being organized around what the mirror, the scale, and the social environment reward. The stomach, liver, pancreas, and intestine did not change. The interpretive frame around them did.

The rise of mass media accelerated that shift because it created a system that could distribute body anxiety at industrial scale. Magazines, television, advertising, and later the internet taught people to see food through the language of slimming, toning, guilt, indulgence, cheating, cleansing, balance, and control. A meal stopped being a package of amino acids, fats, minerals, and carbohydrate structures that would trigger real digestive and hormonal events. It became a personal statement about discipline. Low-fat foods were sold as restraint. Sugar-free foods were sold as moral intelligence. Snack packs, meal replacements, point systems, and portion-controlled products turned metabolism into a consumer ritual. None of this required the public to understand gastric acid, insulin dynamics, satiety hormones, bile release, protein turnover, or micronutrient bioavailability. That was part of the appeal. Diet culture offered a social script that could replace physiology with obedience. Eat this. Avoid that. Count these. Fear those. The body was still doing chemistry underneath the script, but the person was no longer being taught to look there.

This is why diet culture thrives on simplification. It cannot survive if the eater starts asking deeper questions. If the conversation moves to what the body is built from, whether the meal provides enough complete protein, whether the fats are structurally useful, whether blood glucose is being destabilized, whether minerals are being absorbed or bound in the gut lumen, whether satiety is being created or bypassed, the whole enterprise becomes harder to package. Diet culture prefers visible metrics that can be tracked without biological understanding. Weight. inches. calories. meal timing. approved foods. forbidden foods. It reduces the organism to a project of external management because external management is easier to sell than internal literacy. A person can be kept cycling through plans indefinitely if he never learns how the body actually interprets incoming food. Confusion is profitable. Structural understanding is not.

The damage is not only intellectual. It is physiological. Diet culture routinely encourages people to pursue short-term visual outcomes by overriding appetite, underfeeding protein, reducing nutrient density, or building meals around engineered low-calorie products that satisfy the plan more than the organism. A person can become smaller while feeding the body worse. He can improve compliance while worsening satiety. He can follow the rules perfectly while increasing digestive friction, weakening lean tissue maintenance, or creating repeated swings in blood glucose and hunger. The public then interprets failure through a moral frame. I was not disciplined enough. I fell off the wagon. I lost control. But the underlying problem is often mechanical. The food pattern did not fit human biology well enough to remain stable without force. It did not supply enough of what the body needed, or it destabilized signaling in ways that made continued adherence progressively harder. The body is then blamed for resisting a pattern that never matched its requirements in the first place.

Biological understanding begins where diet culture cannot. It begins with the organism instead of the social script. The question becomes what raw materials the body must receive repeatedly in order to preserve structure, stable energy, hormonal coherence, immune function, and tissue repair. It asks how food is actually processed, what digestion can liberate, what reaches the bloodstream, what creates satiety, what causes volatility, and what the body must clear afterward. That shift breaks the emotional hold of diet culture because it replaces morality with mechanism. Food is no longer a badge of virtue or failure. It is an input that either supports the organism cleanly or forces the organism to compensate. Once that becomes clear, the rise of diet culture stops looking like nutritional progress and starts looking like a long detour away from anatomy, chemistry, and common physiological sense.

Weight-Loss Thinking vs Structural Nutrition

Weight-loss thinking begins with reduction. Structural nutrition begins with construction. That difference sounds small until it reaches tissue. In the weight-loss frame, food is judged mainly by how effectively it lowers intake, suppresses appetite for a few hours, reduces scale weight, or creates a measurable deficit between energy consumed and energy expended. The body is treated like stored mass that must be pared down. Structural nutrition starts somewhere else entirely. It starts with the fact that the organism is made of proteins, lipids, minerals, water, and regulated signaling systems that must be maintained continuously whether body fat is rising, falling, or stable. Muscle proteins still have to be rebuilt. Intestinal cells still turn over. Enzymes still degrade and need replacement. Steroid hormones still require cholesterol and adequate metabolic support. Cell membranes still need usable fatty acids. Mitochondria still need substrates and cofactors to produce adenosine triphosphate, or ATP, the immediate energy currency of the cell. A person can lose weight while underfeeding all of that. The scale may approve while the tissues begin paying.

This is why weight-loss thinking so often mistakes visible change for physiological success. Early weight loss is frequently a mixed event composed of glycogen depletion, water loss, reduced gut bulk, less sodium retention, and some degree of true fat loss. Glycogen is the storage form of glucose held in liver and muscle, and it binds water with it. When carbohydrate intake falls or total intake drops sharply, glycogen falls and water leaves with it. The body gets lighter quickly. That rapid shift is real, but it says very little by itself about long-term nutritional adequacy. A person can become smaller on a pattern that is protein-poor, fat-phobic, micronutrient-thin, or digestively irritating.

He can improve a short-term visual metric while weakening satiety, lowering training recovery, shrinking lean mass, reducing mineral intake, and increasing dependency on willpower to stay on plan. Weight-loss thinking rarely stops to ask what was preserved during the loss, what was sacrificed, and what materials are still entering the body in sufficient quantity to keep repair, immunity, endocrine function, and neurological stability intact.

Structural nutrition judges the same meal by a harder standard. Not how little it contributes to body mass, but what it contributes to body structure. Does it deliver complete protein that digestion can liberate into amino acids with high efficiency. Does it provide fats that can be incorporated into membranes, oxidized for steady energy, and used in hormone synthesis. Does it carry minerals in chemically available forms, or are they trapped by binders before they ever reach the absorptive surface of the intestine. Does it create strong satiety through gastric slowing, amino acid signaling, and stable post-meal fuel access, or does it leave the eater lighter on paper but biochemically unfinished. This is where many diet foods collapse. They are designed to satisfy the arithmetic of weight loss while starving the architecture. A low-calorie snack bar may reduce intake compared with a larger meal, yet still arrive as a poor protein source, a weak fat source, a glucose-disrupting carbohydrate source, and a chemically thin package that does little for real tissue maintenance. The number improves. The organism does not.

The hormonal picture makes the difference even sharper. Weight-loss thinking often assumes that the central task is to force less energy into the body. Structural nutrition asks what kind of endocrine environment the food creates once it is eaten. Meals built around adequate protein and supportive fat tend to slow gastric emptying, increase cholecystokinin and peptide YY, provide more durable satiety, and reduce the need for repeated feeding. Meals built around refined carbohydrate and low structural density can do the opposite. They move fast, raise blood glucose quickly, provoke a larger insulin response relative to their structural value, and often return the eater to hunger without having supplied much of what the body actually needed. In that state, the person is told he lacks discipline. The physiology tells a different story. The meal did not finish the job. It delivered energy faster than structure. The body kept asking for materials while the diet program congratulated itself for being light.

This is why structural nutrition is the more serious frame. It does not ignore body composition. It simply refuses to treat body composition as the only question. Fat loss matters, but the route matters too. The body should not have to become weaker, less nourished, more brittle, more inflamed, or more metabolically unstable in order to become leaner. A successful nutritional pattern is one that allows excess stored energy to fall while preserving or improving the quality of the organism losing it. That means adequate amino acids for lean tissue, adequate fats for membranes and hormones, adequate micronutrients for enzymatic work, and foods that digestion can process with high yield and low friction. Weight-loss thinking asks how to make the body smaller. Structural nutrition asks how to make the body better built while allowing unnecessary mass to leave. That is the higher standard, and it is the one this book will use.

Why the Body Is Not Managed by Slogans, Guilt, or Food Morality

The body has no mechanism for moral interpretation. It does not detect whether a meal was virtuous, indulgent, clean, dirty, disciplined, balanced, or a cheat. It detects acids, amino acids, glucose, fatty acids, minerals, osmotic load, mechanical stretch, hormonal signals, and inflammatory stress. Food enters the mouth as matter from the outside world, not as a moral proposition. From there it is chewed, mixed with saliva, exposed to stomach acid, broken apart by enzymes, moved through the intestinal lumen, absorbed across epithelial membranes, routed through the liver, distributed through blood, incorporated into tissue, stored, oxidized, or excreted. That entire sequence is chemical and structural. The stomach does not intensify protein digestion because the meal was earned. The pancreas does not reduce insulin output because the eater feels guilty. The intestine does not increase mineral absorption because the plate matches a wellness ideal. The organism is not governed by emotional language. It is governed by physiological handling.

This matters because slogans are built to override complexity, while digestion depends on it. Eat clean. Everything in moderation. Follow the plan. Make better choices. Avoid bad foods. Respect your body. These phrases can shape behavior, but they do not explain what the body is actually doing once food arrives. A person can follow a slogan perfectly and still eat in a way that destabilizes appetite, underdelivers protein, weakens mineral intake, or floods the bloodstream with rapidly absorbed carbohydrate. Another person can violate the approved language and still give the body dense amino acids, usable fats, fat-soluble vitamins, and stronger satiety. The body does not reward compliance to a phrase. It responds to the nutrient structure, digestion burden, absorption profile, and hormonal consequence of the meal itself. That is why slogan-based eating so often produces confusion. The language feels clear. The biology underneath it remains unexamined.

Guilt fails for the same reason. Guilt is a psychological event, not a digestive one. It may alter stress signaling through the nervous system, and chronic stress can certainly affect appetite, gastric function, bowel motility, and blood glucose regulation. But guilt does not transform low-value food into nourishment, and it does not turn nutrient-dense food into poison. It does not change whether a protein is complete, whether bile is needed to emulsify fat, whether phytic acid binds zinc in the gut, or whether a refined carbohydrate load drives a rapid insulin surge. Guilt often enters nutrition as a substitute for understanding. The eater is taught to feel morally defective for hunger, cravings, loss of control, or weight regain, when the real problem may be that the food pattern was structurally weak and hormonally unstable. A person who is repeatedly underfed in protein, pushed toward low-satiety foods, or exposed to large swings in blood glucose does not need a lecture in virtue. He needs a better biological input.

Food morality creates another distortion by assigning ethical value to categories that the body experiences very differently than the culture describes them. A food can be praised because it is plant-based, low-fat, natural, whole grain, or lightly processed, yet still create digestive friction, unstable appetite, weak structural nutrition, or a poor net yield once absorption and tissue use are counted. Another food can be treated with suspicion because it is rich, fatty, or animal-derived while supplying exactly what the organism needs in concentrated, absorbable form. The moral frame blocks real accounting because it protects appearances. It allows reputation to stand in for outcome. But the body keeps a harder ledger. What digestion released. What stayed bound. What crossed into blood. What reached tissue. What burdened clearance. What remained useful after the full event was complete. That is the only moral language the organism recognizes, if moral language is to be used at all. Input and consequence. Exposure and result.

Once this is understood, nutrition becomes quieter and more exact. The eater no longer has to ask whether a food feels righteous or shameful.

The better question is what kind of physiological event it creates. Does it provide complete amino acids for repair. Does it deliver fats that support membranes, satiety, and steady fuel access. Does it create a manageable glucose response. Does it carry minerals in forms that remain available through digestion. Does it nourish without excessive burden. That shift removes a great deal of emotional theater from food and replaces it with something more demanding but far more honest. The body is not waiting to approve your intentions. It is processing what you gave it.

Moving from Rules to Biological Principles

Rules are attractive because they make food feel manageable from the outside. Eat every three hours. Do not eat after seven. Always eat breakfast. Never snack. Avoid red meat. Choose whole grains. Limit saturated fat. Count your calories. Hit your macros. The rule gives the eater something clear to do, and for a while that clarity can feel like progress. But rules only tell a person how to behave. They do not tell him what the body is doing in response. A rule can accidentally help because it reduces refined carbohydrates, increases protein, lengthens the gap between insulin surges, lowers exposure to hyper-palatable processed food, or improves digestive rhythm. But once the rule is detached from the mechanism that made it useful, it becomes fragile. The person follows the behavior without understanding the organism. That is why the same rule can appear to work for one person, fail for another, and collapse completely when context changes. Biology is still running underneath it, but the eater has been taught to obey the surface pattern instead of reading the internal event.

Biological principles start at a deeper level. They begin with what the body must repeatedly receive and what the body is forced to manage after every meal. Protein is not important because a diet trend says to prioritize it. It is important because enzymes, transport proteins, muscle tissue, immune molecules, connective tissue, and much of the body's repair machinery are built from amino acids, and those amino acids must arrive in sufficient quantity and in usable balance. Fat is not valuable because it fits a low-carb philosophy. It is valuable because the body uses fatty acids and cholesterol to build membranes, produce steroid hormones, absorb fat-soluble vitamins, and maintain stable access to fuel. Carbohydrate is not good or bad because a rulebook approves or condemns it. It is a fuel signal whose biological effect depends on form, quantity, digestive speed, and the metabolic condition of the person eating it. Once food is understood at that level, the question changes. The eater stops asking what the rule says and starts asking what the meal supplies, what it disrupts, and what it costs the body to process.

That shift matters because rules often confuse compliance with nourishment. A person can follow a perfectly clean-looking diet and still underfeed structural needs if protein is too low, fat is too restricted, or food choice is built around ideas rather than usable nutrient density. Another person can break several fashionable rules and still feed the body better because the food actually delivers complete amino acids, stable fats, bioavailable minerals, and stronger satiety. Biological principles force this kind of honesty. They ask whether stomach acid can denature the incoming proteins effectively, whether bile flow is adequate to emulsify dietary fat, whether the intestine can absorb the nutrients in question, whether blood glucose is rising in a controlled range or surging fast enough to require aggressive insulin handling, whether minerals remain soluble in the gut lumen or are being trapped by binding compounds before absorption can occur. A rule never reaches that level. It tells the person when to eat or what category to avoid. A principle explains what the body is trying to accomplish and how a food either supports that work or complicates it.

Once the reader begins thinking in principles, flexibility increases while confusion drops. The person no longer needs a separate commandment for every situation because the underlying logic becomes portable. If protein supports structural repair and satiety, then meals built around adequate protein make sense in many contexts without needing a slogan attached to them. If refined carbohydrate creates rapid glucose delivery with weak structural value, then its effects become easier to predict without relying on a trendy prohibition. If certain foods create digestive friction, unstable appetite, or poor net nutrient yield, then reducing them becomes a rational biological decision rather than an act of dietary purity. This is where nutrition becomes more adult, more exact, and less theatrical. The eater is no longer being managed by rules handed down from outside. He is learning to see the organism from the inside and choose food according to what that organism actually needs.

Chapter 3

The Body Is Not a Calorie Spreadsheet

The calorie model did not begin inside human physiology. It began in physics. A calorie is a unit of heat, a way of measuring how much thermal energy is released when a substance is burned. That origin matters because it shaped the kind of question early nutrition science learned to ask. Instead of beginning with digestion, hormonal signaling, tissue repair, or cellular fuel selection, the model began with combustion. Food was treated as a measurable energy source, and the practical problem became how much potential heat it contained. In laboratory terms, this was straightforward. A food sample could be placed in a bomb calorimeter, a sealed device that burns the sample completely and measures the heat released into surrounding water. The output was a number. That number could then be used to compare foods by energetic potential. Fat yielded more heat than carbohydrate or protein. Sugars and starches yielded less. The logic was clean, quantifiable, and attractive. It gave scientists and later public health institutions a simple way to talk about food as fuel. But the body does not run food through open flame. It does not incinerate a meal into heat and call the job done. It digests, absorbs, sorts, stores, oxidizes, and builds. The calorie entered nutrition by way of measurement convenience, not by way of biological completeness.

Once that heat model was imported into nutrition, it offered something powerful to researchers and policy makers. It made food easier to count. This mattered enormously in eras concerned with famine, military provisioning, industrial labor, and later obesity. If food could be reduced to units of energy, then diets could be planned in numerical terms. Rations could be designed. Weight change could be described as an energy problem. Public guidance could be simplified into intake and expenditure. This framework gained more force when early twentieth century nutrition science was still developing tools for understanding micronutrients, endocrine regulation, mitochondrial function, and tissue-specific fuel handling. Heat accounting looked objective. It appeared universal. It also fit the industrial mindset of the time, which preferred systems that could be measured, standardized, and scaled. The more food was reduced to a number, the easier it became to compare one eating pattern with another without entering the messy interior of the organism. A growing child, a manual laborer, and an office worker could all be discussed through the same accounting language. The body began to be framed less as a living construction project and more as an energy budget.

That shift created a model with real usefulness but severe limitations. Yes, the body must obey thermodynamics. It cannot create energy from nothing. But thermodynamics does not tell you how the organism handles different incoming nutrients, how much energy is lost in digestion and conversion, how strongly insulin responds to one meal versus another, whether amino acids are being used to build tissue or burned because the diet is imbalanced, or whether a food creates strong satiety or drives repeated feeding. Protein, fat, and carbohydrate do not enter metabolism as interchangeable tokens. Protein arrives as amino acid chains that must be denatured by hydrochloric acid, cut apart by proteases, absorbed, and then directed toward enzyme synthesis, immune proteins, structural repair, neurotransmitter precursors, or glucose production when necessary. Fat arrives as hydrophobic lipid structures that require bile acids for emulsification, pancreatic lipase for hydrolysis, micelle formation for transport through the aqueous gut environment, and lymphatic packaging into chylomicrons before wider circulation. Carbohydrate often arrives with very different kinetics, especially when refined. It can move rapidly, appear quickly as glucose in the bloodstream, and trigger a strong insulin signal that changes whether incoming fuel is oxidized immediately or pushed toward storage. The calorimeter does not see any of this. It sees burnable material. The organism sees a sequence of regulatory decisions.

The calorie model therefore became dominant not because it fully described human metabolism, but because it offered a simple external abstraction of something much more complex. Once that abstraction became culturally embedded, public nutrition drifted toward arithmetic. Eat less, move more. Burn more than you consume. Manage the ledger. That language survived because it was easy to teach and easy to moralize. It made body weight look like a math problem with a character component. But the body is not managed from the outside by a bookkeeping script. It is managed from the inside by hormones, enzymes, transport proteins, organ priorities, nutrient sufficiency, and the physical chemistry of digestion and absorption. Two foods can contain the same measured energy and still create profoundly different biological events because the body is not reading the label as a heat total. It is reading amino acid availability, glucose delivery speed, fatty acid type, micronutrient density, osmotic load, fiber burden, and satiety signaling. The calorie model survived because it is numerically tidy. Human physiology is not tidy. It is layered.

This is why the calorie model must be placed in its proper historical position. It is a tool, not a governing theory of life. It can estimate energetic potential. It can help explain why chronic excess intake eventually accumulates as stored mass. It cannot tell you whether a food nourishes well, whether it supplies structural material, whether it destabilizes appetite, whether it burdens digestion, or whether the body will remain biologically compatible with that intake pattern over time. The mistake was not measuring energy. The mistake was allowing a heat unit imported from physics to become the dominant language for a living organism built from tissue, membranes, enzymes, hormones, and regulated fuel systems. Once nutrition is returned to physiology, the calorie can keep its limited place. It simply loses its throne.

Why Heat Measurement Is Not Metabolism

Heat measurement treats food as if its meaning were exhausted once it burns. That is the central problem. A bomb calorimeter places food inside a sealed chamber, ignites it, and measures how much thermal energy is released during complete combustion. The result is a clean number, but it is a number produced by destruction, not by life. The body does not incinerate steak, fruit, butter, or starch in an oxygen-rich steel vessel and convert the whole event into heat. It subjects food to chewing, acid exposure, enzymatic cleavage, membrane transport, intracellular processing, organ-level sorting, hormone signaling, mitochondrial oxidation, tissue construction, and waste disposal. Heat may be generated during those processes, because living metabolism does release heat, but heat release is a byproduct of the system, not the system itself. Metabolism is the managed extraction, transformation, and use of nutrients inside a living structure. A calorimeter sees burnable matter. The body sees amino acids, fatty acids, glucose, minerals, cofactors, osmotic loads, digestive burdens, and signaling instructions.

That difference begins in the gut. When food enters the body, it does not become metabolically relevant until digestion has made its contents accessible. Protein must be denatured by hydrochloric acid, unfolded so peptide bonds become accessible, then cut by proteases into peptides and amino acids that can cross the intestinal lining. Fat has to be emulsified by bile acids because it does not mix with the watery environment of the intestine. Pancreatic lipase must hydrolyze triglycerides into fatty acids and monoglycerides, which then have to be packaged for transport through the lymphatic system. Carbohydrate has to be broken into absorbable sugars and then handled through tightly regulated glucose transport and insulin signaling. None of this is captured by heat measurement. The calorie model assumes the energy in the food is what matters most. Physiology asks a prior question. Can the body actually access the material cleanly, and what regulatory state does that access create. A food can contain measurable energy and still deliver it in a way that destabilizes blood glucose, weakens satiety, burdens digestion, or contributes little to structure.

The body is also not interested in energy alone. It is trying to preserve architecture. Amino acids are not important because they can be burned. They are important because the body uses them to build enzymes, transport proteins, immune molecules, connective tissue, muscle fibers, neurotransmitter precursors, and countless other structures. Fatty acids are not just energy reserves. They become part of cell membranes, influence membrane fluidity, participate in signaling cascades, support steroid hormone production, and help carry fat-soluble vitamins into the body. Minerals do not function as calories at all, yet they are essential for electrical gradients, enzyme activity, oxygen transport, and structural integrity. The calorie model cannot explain any of this because it flattens food into a potential heat total. A bomb calorimeter can tell you that protein, fat, and carbohydrate all yield energy when burned. It cannot tell you that one food may rebuild tissue while another mainly floods the bloodstream with rapidly available glucose, or that one nutrient may be essential for membrane structure while another is largely a fast fuel signal.

Metabolism is also regulated, and regulation is exactly what heat measurement leaves out. The body does not passively receive energy. It decides what to do with incoming material through hormones, transporters, enzyme activity, and organ priorities. Insulin rises in response to glucose and changes fuel partitioning by pushing nutrients toward storage and cellular uptake. Glucagon, cortisol, thyroid hormones, leptin, ghrelin, cholecystokinin, and many other signals continuously alter hunger, satiety, substrate selection, and energy access. The liver directs some nutrients toward glycogen storage, others toward oxidation, others toward synthesis, and still others toward detoxification and excretion. The mitochondrion does not simply burn nutrients indiscriminately. It processes substrates through specific pathways such as beta-oxidation, glycolysis, the citric acid cycle, and oxidative phosphorylation. These pathways differ in speed, byproducts, regulatory control, and tissue preference. Heat measurement sees none of that hierarchy. It cannot tell the difference between a meal that creates stable access to fuel and one that produces a rapid spike followed by a crash. It cannot tell the difference between nutrients that support satiety and those that drive repeated intake.

This is why two foods with similar calorie values can produce very different biological outcomes. A meal of eggs and beef may generate strong satiety, slower gastric emptying, sustained amino acid availability, stable fuel access through fat oxidation, and meaningful structural nourishment. A meal of refined cereal and sweetened yogurt may deliver a comparable heat value on paper while creating a much faster glucose rise, a stronger insulin response relative to its structural value, weaker satiety, and a quicker return of hunger. The calories may look similar when reduced to combustion math. The metabolic event is not similar at all. One pattern feeds tissue and stabilizes signaling. The other pushes rapid energy through the system with far less structural payoff. The difference is not philosophical. It is physiological.

Heat measurement can estimate potential energy. That is all. Metabolism is the living choreography that determines whether food becomes structure, stable fuel, stored energy, waste, inflammatory burden, or repeated hunger. The body is not a furnace with opinions. It is a regulated organism with tissues to maintain and signals to interpret. That is why heat measurement is not metabolism. It measures what a food can release when destroyed. Metabolism determines what a body can do with it while alive.

Hormones, Nutrient Signaling, and Energy Partitioning

The body does not manage incoming food by counting calories and then filing them into a neutral storage ledger. It manages food through hormonal interpretation. Every meal arrives as a set of chemical signals, and those signals tell the organism what kind of metabolic environment it is dealing with. Glucose rising in the bloodstream means one thing. Amino acids appearing after protein digestion mean another. Fatty acids entering circulation through chylomicrons, the lipid transport particles formed after intestinal fat absorption, mean something else again. Hormones translate those signals into action. They determine whether energy is used immediately, stored for later, released from reserves, or directed toward repair and construction. This is what energy partitioning actually means. It is the body's decision process for where incoming fuel and structural material go once they have crossed into the internal environment.

Insulin sits at the center of this process because it is one of the primary hormones that tells tissues that energy is abundant and available for uptake. When blood glucose rises after carbohydrate digestion, pancreatic beta cells release insulin into circulation. Insulin then binds to receptors on cells and changes their behavior. It increases glucose uptake in muscle and adipose tissue, supports glycogen formation in liver and muscle, suppresses lipolysis, the release of stored fat from adipose tissue, and pushes the body toward storage and fed-state handling. That does not make insulin evil. It makes insulin directional. It is a traffic hormone. It tells the organism that incoming fuel is present and that storage, containment, and distribution need to happen. The problem begins when that signal is driven hard and repeatedly by meals that deliver glucose rapidly, especially when those meals are structurally weak in protein and micronutrients and do little to create durable satiety. In that environment, energy partitioning tilts toward repeated storage pressure while appetite may remain incompletely satisfied.

Protein creates a different signaling pattern. When dietary protein is digested and amino acids enter the bloodstream, the body does not simply interpret them as fuel. It interprets them as raw material for repair, enzyme synthesis, immune function, transport proteins, and tissue maintenance. Amino acids stimulate insulin to some degree, but they also stimulate glucagon and activate pathways related to protein synthesis, particularly when essential amino acids such as leucine are present in sufficient quantity. The result is not the same metabolic instruction as a refined carbohydrate load. A protein-rich meal tells the body that structural material has arrived. It supports repair and maintenance while also contributing to satiety through gastric slowing, digestive hormone release, and the gradual appearance of amino acids in circulation. The hormonal meaning of that meal is different because the nutrient signal is different. This is why calories alone do not explain the event. The same nominal energy value can produce very different partitioning decisions depending on whether it arrived as glucose, amino acids, or fat.

Fat sends yet another message. Dietary fat, once emulsified by bile, hydrolyzed by pancreatic lipase, absorbed through the intestine, and packaged into chylomicrons, enters circulation in a way that is slower and more extended than glucose. It does not usually provoke the same rapid insulin excursion that refined carbohydrate does. Instead, it contributes to satiety, slows gastric emptying, and provides a dense source of fuel that can be oxidized over longer periods of time. Fatty acids can be directed toward immediate oxidation, stored in adipose tissue, incorporated into cell membranes, or used in the synthesis of signaling molecules and steroid hormones depending on the organism's state. Again, the body is not reading a calorie number. It is reading the chemical form of the incoming substrate and then assigning it to pathways according to need, hormonal context, and current fuel availability. Energy partitioning is therefore not a simple matter of excess or deficit. It is a regulated sorting process shaped by the nutrient composition of the meal and the metabolic condition of the person eating it.

This is where the larger endocrine network becomes impossible to ignore. Insulin is only one part of the system. Glucagon helps mobilize stored fuel when incoming glucose is low. Leptin reflects longer-term energy storage in adipose tissue and influences appetite and energy expenditure. Ghrelin rises before meals and helps drive hunger. Cholecystokinin and peptide YY respond to protein and fat digestion and help generate satiety. Cortisol can shift fuel use under stress and raise glucose availability. Thyroid hormones influence the overall speed and intensity of metabolic activity. None of these signals act in isolation. They form a living control system that interprets food and then allocates energy and resources accordingly. A diet that destabilizes these signals can push a person toward repeated hunger, erratic energy, excessive storage, poor recovery, and rising metabolic friction even if the calorie math looks respectable on paper. A diet that aligns with them can make appetite calmer, energy steadier, and tissue maintenance more reliable without theatrical restriction.

Once hormones and nutrient signaling are placed back into the story, nutrition stops looking like arithmetic and starts looking like biological traffic control. The body is constantly deciding what to burn, what to build, what to store, and what to release. Those decisions are shaped by the form, speed, and structural value of incoming food. A meal rich in complete protein and supportive fat creates a different endocrine environment from one built around refined carbohydrate and weak satiety. That difference is not theoretical. It determines whether energy remains stable or volatile, whether tissues receive useful material or mainly disposable fuel, and whether stored energy becomes accessible or remains locked away behind repeated insulin pressure. This is why energy partitioning matters. The food is not just entering the body. It is telling the body what kind of metabolic world it thinks it is living in.

Why Two Foods With Equal Calories Can Produce Very Different Biological Outcomes

Equal calories do not mean equal biological effect because the body does not receive food as abstract energy. It receives food as structure, chemistry, and timing. A calorie is only a unit of potential heat, not a description of what the digestive tract had to do, what hormones were triggered, what nutrients were liberated, what crossed the intestinal membrane, what tissues could actually use, and what remained as burden or waste after the event was over. Two foods can carry the same measured energy and still place the body in completely different metabolic states because the organism is not reading the label as a number. It is reading the incoming material as amino acids, fatty acids, glucose, minerals, water content, osmotic load, fiber structure, and signaling information. A meal of eggs and beef and a meal of sweetened cereal and fruit juice may be matched on paper for energy, yet one arrives with dense protein, usable fat, slower gastric emptying, stronger satiety signaling, and direct structural value, while the other delivers rapidly absorbable sugar, weak tissue-building value, faster glucose entry, a larger insulin demand, and a quicker return of hunger. The heat total may look similar. The physiological event is not similar at all.

The difference begins in digestion. Protein-rich foods have to be denatured by stomach acid, cleaved by proteases, and absorbed as amino acids and small peptides. Fat has to be emulsified by bile, hydrolyzed by lipase, assembled into transport particles, and delivered through lymphatic circulation. These processes take time, and that time matters because it changes the rate at which nutrients appear in the bloodstream. A refined carbohydrate food often requires far less digestive work before glucose begins entering circulation. The faster that happens, the faster pancreatic insulin secretion must rise to manage it. That shifts the entire post-meal environment. One food produces a slower, broader release of nutrients into the system. The other creates a sharper fuel surge that has to be contained quickly. This is why a calorie from a fast sugar source and a calorie from a protein-and-fat source do not feel the same, do not regulate appetite the same way, and do not partition energy the same way.

Hormonal signaling deepens the separation. A food that produces rapid glucose absorption drives a different endocrine response than a food dominated by protein and fat. Insulin rises more aggressively when blood glucose rises quickly. That insulin signal changes fuel partitioning by driving glucose into tissues, promoting glycogen storage when capacity remains, and pushing excess energy toward storage when immediate use is limited. Protein, by contrast, brings amino acids into circulation that support tissue repair, enzyme synthesis, immune function, and muscle protein synthesis while also stimulating satiety hormones such as cholecystokinin and peptide YY. Fat contributes to slower gastric emptying and more sustained energy delivery. These meals do not merely differ in composition. They tell the body different stories about incoming resources. One says fast fuel has arrived and must be managed immediately. Another says structural material and stable fuel have arrived and can support repair and satiety. Equal calories do not erase that signaling difference.

The quality of what is delivered also matters because the body is not trying to meet an energy target alone. It is trying to maintain structure. Cells need membrane lipids. Tissues need amino acids. Enzymes need mineral cofactors. Hormones need raw material. If a food delivers energy but few of the molecules required for tissue maintenance, the body may still be energetically fed and biologically undernourished at the same time. This is one reason processed foods can promote continued eating even when calorie intake is already high. They solve the short-term fuel problem poorly and often fail to solve the structural problem at all. A nutrient-dense food can shut appetite down more effectively because it gives the organism something closer to what it was actually asking for. The body is not searching for calories in the abstract. It is searching for usable material.

This is why equal calorie comparisons become misleading when they are treated as the final word. They flatten digestive speed, nutrient density, bioavailability, hormonal response, satiety, and tissue consequence into one number and then pretend the biological work is finished. It is not. The real comparison must ask what the body extracted, how rapidly it appeared, what it signaled, what it built, what it stored, and what it left the organism needing afterward. Two foods may enter with the same theoretical energy. One may leave the body calmer, better fed, and less interested in eating again soon. The other may leave it unstable, incompletely nourished, and searching for the next input. That is not a minor difference. That is the difference between arithmetic and physiology.

Why Appetite Is Often a Nutrient Problem, Not a Math Problem

Appetite is usually treated as if it were a bookkeeping error. The person ate too much, failed to count accurately, underestimated portions, or lacked enough discipline to maintain the intended deficit. That frame sounds clean, but it starts too late and explains too little. The body does not generate hunger by performing calorie arithmetic in the abstract and then punishing people for weak character. Hunger emerges from tissue need, digestive signaling, fuel access, hormonal state, and the degree to which the last meal actually supplied usable material. A person can consume large amounts of energy and still remain biologically unsatisfied if the food delivered fast fuel without enough complete protein, supportive fat, minerals, or durable satiety signals. In that situation, appetite is not evidence of mathematical incompetence. It is evidence that the organism is still looking for something.

The digestive sequence makes this visible. A meal rich in protein and fat tends to stay in the stomach longer, stimulate stronger release of satiety hormones such as cholecystokinin and peptide YY, and deliver amino acids and fatty acids over a longer time window. That slows the return of hunger because the body is receiving both structural material and a steadier fuel supply. A meal built from refined carbohydrate often behaves differently. It can empty from the stomach more quickly, break down rapidly into absorbable sugars, raise blood glucose sharply, and provoke a larger insulin response relative to its structural value. Blood glucose is then contained, sometimes quickly, while the deeper nutritional problem remains partly unsolved. The body received energy.

It did not necessarily receive enough of what it needed to repair tissue, stabilize satiety, and reduce the drive to continue seeking food. Hunger returns, and the eater is told to focus on willpower. The physiology is telling a simpler story. The meal finished poorly.

Protein is central here because amino acids are not optional background nutrients. They are the raw material for enzymes, transport proteins, muscle tissue, immune molecules, connective tissue, and countless repair processes. The body does not keep a large storage warehouse of free amino acids the way it stores fat. It depends on repeated intake. If meals are low in complete protein, appetite can remain elevated because the body still has unresolved structural demand. This is one reason people can overconsume processed foods and still feel strangely unfinished. They have met an energy target without meeting a construction target. The same problem appears with fat. Dietary fat slows gastric emptying, supports stable post-meal energy, helps with absorption of fat-soluble vitamins, and contributes to the endocrine environment that tells the body it is fed. When fat is chronically stripped out and replaced with low-satiety carbohydrate volume, appetite often becomes louder, not quieter. The eater is being under-signaled and under-supplied at the same time.

Micronutrients matter as well, though they are easier to ignore because they do not announce themselves as clearly as protein. Minerals and vitamins function as cofactors in enzyme systems, energy production, oxygen handling, nerve signaling, and tissue maintenance. A diet dominated by refined foods can deliver substantial calories while remaining thin in usable minerals and other regulatory compounds. The person may not consciously crave zinc, magnesium, iron, or B vitamins by name, but the body still detects incomplete nourishment through altered energy, weak satiety, poor recovery, and persistent food-seeking. Appetite in that context is not always a direct request for more calories. It is often the body pushing for another chance to obtain what the previous meal failed to supply.

This is why calorie math so often breaks down in real life. It assumes appetite should obey the plan as long as the number is correct. But appetite is not designed to defend a spreadsheet. It is designed to protect the organism. If food quality is poor, if protein is inadequate, if fat is too restricted, if blood sugar is unstable, if meals are built around rapidly absorbed energy with weak structural payoff, hunger will often rise regardless of what the calorie target says. The person then experiences this as personal failure because the culture has trained him to interpret appetite morally. Biology offers a harder but more accurate interpretation. Hunger is frequently the downstream voice of unresolved nutritional demand, unstable fuel handling, or incomplete satiety signaling.

Once appetite is seen this way, the strategy changes. The goal is no longer to overpower hunger with rules alone. The goal is to feed the body in a way that reduces the biological reason for hunger to stay active. That means meals with enough complete protein to satisfy structural demand, enough supportive fat to stabilize digestion and energy delivery, and enough nutrient density to reduce the body's need to keep searching. Appetite can certainly be distorted by habit, reward circuitry, and hyper-palatable food engineering, but even then the repair still begins with better input. The body is easier to live with when it is actually being fed. Hunger is not always a math problem. Very often it is a signal that the organism is still waiting for real nourishment.

Chapter 4

Food as Biological Input

Food enters the body as external matter, but once digestion begins it stops being a menu item and becomes biological input. That input does three kinds of work whether the eater understands it or not. It supplies structure, it supplies energy, and it supplies signals. Modern nutrition usually isolates one of these and treats it as the whole story. Calories reduce food to energy. vitamin language reduces food to nutrient presence. diet culture reduces food to behavioral control. The body does none of that. It breaks food down into usable parts and then asks three hard questions at once. What can be built from this. What can be burned from this. What instructions does this send to the endocrine system, the digestive tract, the liver, the brain, and the cell. A meal that looks acceptable from one angle can fail badly from another. A food can be energetic and structurally poor. It can be rich on a label and weak in real delivery. It can fill the stomach while sending unstable signals that drive more eating later. This is why food has to be understood as a three-part biological event rather than a number or a category.

The structural role of food is the least appreciated and the most important. The body is not made from calories. It is made from tissue. Muscles, enzymes, transport proteins, immune molecules, connective fibers, cell membranes, bone matrix, steroid hormones, neurotransmitter precursors. All of these require raw material. Protein provides amino acids that the body uses to rebuild and maintain much of its internal machinery. Fat provides fatty acids and cholesterol that contribute to membrane architecture, hormone synthesis, nervous system function, and the absorption of fat-soluble vitamins. Minerals provide electrical charge, structural support, and enzyme cofactors. If these materials do not arrive in sufficient quantity and usable form, the body does not stop needing them. It compensates. It breaks down tissue, slows processes, weakens repair, alters signaling, and keeps appetite active in the hope that better material will arrive later. This is why a diet can be high in energy and still leave the body underbuilt. The organism is asking for parts, not just fuel.

Energy is the second role, but even here the body is more selective than most nutrition language admits. It does not simply ask how much energy entered. It asks what form that energy arrived in, how quickly it can be accessed, and what hormonal state that fuel creates. Carbohydrate often provides rapid fuel through glucose. Fat provides slower, more durable energy and can support longer periods of stable fuel access. Protein can be burned when necessary, but that is not its primary value. The body would rather use amino acids to build and maintain than waste them as expensive fuel. This means the energy role of food is not neutral. A rapidly absorbed carbohydrate meal can push the body into one metabolic state, marked by sharp glucose entry and stronger insulin handling, while a meal built around protein and fat can push it into another, marked by slower gastric emptying, steadier fuel release, and stronger satiety. Both meals may contain measurable energy. They do not produce the same energetic experience inside the organism.

The signaling role of food is where the model becomes impossible to ignore. Every meal tells the body something about the environment. A fast sugar load says quick fuel has arrived and must be managed immediately. A protein-rich meal says structural material is available for repair and synthesis. A fat-rich meal says longer-duration fuel and membrane material have arrived and digestion should slow down accordingly. The digestive tract responds through acid secretion, bile release, enzyme output, and motility changes. The pancreas responds through insulin and glucagon. The intestine responds through satiety hormones such as cholecystokinin and peptide YY. The liver changes fuel handling, storage, and distribution. The brain changes appetite and energy perception. Food is therefore not simply going into the system. It is instructing the system. This is why identical calorie totals can behave so differently. The body is not just receiving heat potential. It is receiving instructions about storage, access, construction, and urgency.

Once food is understood in these three dimensions, many modern confusions begin to clear. A highly processed snack may be dense in energy while weak in structure and disorderly in signaling. It may flood the bloodstream with quick fuel, create a short burst of reward, and still leave the organism looking for amino acids, minerals, and real satiety. A piece of meat with natural fat may provide strong structure, stable energy, and a signaling pattern that quiets appetite because the body recognizes that meaningful material has arrived. The difference is not philosophical. It is mechanical. Food is never just one thing inside the body. It is always structure, energy, and signaling at the same time. The only question is whether those three functions are working together in a way that supports the organism or pulling it in opposite directions.

Protein, Fat, Carbohydrate, and Micronutrients as Biological Instructions

The body does not receive macronutrients and micronutrients as neutral inventory. It receives them as instructions about what kind of work can be done next. Protein tells the organism that structural material has arrived. Fat tells it that stable fuel, membrane components, and lipid-based signaling substrates are available. Carbohydrate tells it that rapidly accessible glucose has entered circulation or will enter shortly. Micronutrients tell enzyme systems whether they have the cofactors required to keep reactions moving. This is the level at which food becomes real. The meal is no longer a cuisine, a preference, or a label. It is a packet of instructions delivered into a digestive and endocrine system that must decide, in real time, what to build, what to burn, what to store, and what to postpone. If those instructions are incomplete, distorted, or contradictory, the body does not solve that problem by optimism. It compensates through altered hunger, altered storage, altered energy, and slower repair.

Protein is the clearest structural instruction because amino acids are the raw material from which much of the body is built and rebuilt. Once dietary protein is denatured by stomach acid, cut by proteases, and absorbed through the intestinal lining, the appearance of amino acids in circulation signals that repair can proceed. Enzymes can be synthesized. Muscle proteins can be maintained. Immune cells can build antibodies and signaling molecules. Connective tissue can be renewed. Amino acids such as leucine also act as direct nutrient signals, telling cells that sufficient substrate exists for protein synthesis to move forward. This is why protein is not simply a source of calories. It is a message about structural sufficiency. When protein intake is too low, the instruction changes. The body begins rationing, recycling, and breaking down tissue to cover essential needs. Appetite may remain active because the structural request was not actually met, even if energy intake looked adequate on paper.

Fat sends a different kind of instruction. It tells the body that a slower, denser, more stable fuel source has arrived and that lipid-dependent processes can be supported. Fatty acids can be oxidized for energy, incorporated into cell membranes, stored for later use, or converted into signaling molecules that influence inflammation, vascular tone, and cellular communication. Cholesterol and lipid substrates can be directed toward steroid hormone synthesis. Fat in the gut also changes digestive behavior. It slows gastric emptying, stimulates cholecystokinin, and increases bile release from the gallbladder, all of which alter satiety and nutrient handling. The presence of dietary fat therefore says more than fuel is available. It says digestion should slow down, absorption of fat-soluble vitamins can proceed, membrane material is present, and the body can shift toward a more sustained energy pattern. Remove fat chronically and that instruction weakens. The organism may still receive calories, but it loses part of the signal for durability, satiety, and lipid-based maintenance.

Carbohydrate is a faster and more conditional instruction. When carbohydrate is digested into glucose and absorbed, the body interprets that as the arrival of quickly accessible fuel. Insulin rises, tissues increase glucose uptake, liver and muscle replenish glycogen when there is room, and excess energy may be pushed toward storage when immediate demand is low. This can be useful in the right context. Glucose is a legitimate fuel, and some tissues depend on it to varying degrees. But carbohydrate is also a more unstable instruction when delivered rapidly and repeatedly in refined form. A large glucose pulse says urgent fuel is present now. It does not necessarily say that structural needs have been met. That is why a carbohydrate-heavy meal can resolve a short-term energy gap while doing little for tissue repair or durable satiety. The body may be fed in one dimension and still underinformed in another. This is where the mistake of calorie thinking becomes obvious. Carbohydrate, protein, and fat do not send the same message even when they contribute measurable energy. The endocrine response, digestive timing, and downstream tissue effect are different because the instructions are different.

Micronutrients operate more quietly, but their instructions run through nearly every part of metabolism. Magnesium, zinc, iron, copper, selenium, iodine, the B vitamins, vitamins A, D, E, and K. These are not decorative extras riding along beside the macros. They function as enzyme cofactors, redox partners, electron carriers, structural minerals, and regulatory molecules that determine whether the larger instructions from protein, fat, and carbohydrate can actually be executed. A body may receive amino acids, but without adequate micronutrient support it cannot run protein synthesis, oxidative metabolism, detoxification, oxygen transport, thyroid hormone production, or antioxidant defense at full capacity. This is why micronutrient deficiency can show up as fatigue, weak recovery, poor appetite regulation, poor temperature regulation, low resilience, or diffuse metabolic inefficiency rather than as one dramatic symptom. The instruction was present, but the machinery that carries it out was underpowered. In practical terms, this means foods have to be judged not just by what they contain, but by whether they deliver the complete set of signals and cofactors required for those contents to become biological action.

Once food is understood this way, the meal stops looking like a simple pile of calories and starts looking like a control panel. Protein says build and repair. Fat says sustain, stabilize, and supply membranes. Carbohydrate says fast fuel is here, manage it. Micronutrients say the machinery has what it needs or it does not. That is how the body reads food. Not as a label. Not as a morality play. Not as a dietary identity. As instructions. The quality of those instructions determines whether the organism moves toward stability or compensation.

Why Food Quality Matters More Than Abstract Calorie Totals

Food quality matters because the body does not live on energy alone. It lives on what that energy arrives with, how that energy is packaged, how quickly it is delivered, what tissues it can support, and what physiological cost is attached to extracting and handling it. Abstract calorie totals flatten all of that into a single number and then pretend the important work has been done. It has not. A calorie tells you only that a food contains potential heat energy. It does not tell you whether the food carries complete protein, usable fats, bioavailable minerals, fat-soluble vitamins, or a chemical structure that digestion can process efficiently. It does not tell you whether blood glucose will rise slowly or violently, whether satiety hormones will engage strongly or weakly, whether the intestine will absorb the nutrients cleanly, or whether the liver and kidneys will be left with manageable work or added burden. A food can be low in calories and still be nutritionally trivial. Another can be calorie-dense and yet deliver exactly the amino acids, lipids, and micronutrients the organism has been waiting for. The body is not trying to win a math contest. It is trying to stay built, fed, and regulated.

This becomes obvious the moment food is judged by net biological yield instead of paper energy. Two foods can supply similar calories while producing opposite results in tissue. A processed snack built from refined flour, industrial oils, flavor systems, and added sugar may deliver energy rapidly while contributing little to structural repair and weak satiety. It is easy to digest in the narrow sense that glucose and fat can be absorbed, but that is not the same as nourishing well. The fuel arrives quickly, the hormonal response is sharp, and the eater may be left hungry again because the meal did not solve the deeper problem of nutrient sufficiency. A meal built from eggs, meat, dairy, or other nutrient-dense whole foods may contain equal or greater calories, yet it delivers complete amino acids, more stable fats, stronger satiety, and a richer micronutrient environment for enzyme systems, membrane maintenance, immune function, and tissue turnover. The numbers may not flatter it. The biology does.

Food quality also matters because digestion is not free. The body pays for every meal with acid production, bile release, enzyme secretion, transport work, and excretory cleanup. Better foods tend to justify that cost. They give the body material that can be retained and used. Poorer foods often increase the workload while delivering weak return. A plant food may carry minerals on a nutrition label but bind them with phytate or oxalate before absorption. A fortified cereal may look nutritionally improved on the box while still functioning as rapidly absorbed starch with thin structural value. A low-fat product may reduce calorie density while also reducing satiety and fat-soluble vitamin handling. Quality is not a luxury category layered on top of calories. It is the question of whether the organism is being fed intelligently or merely loaded with disposable energy.

This is why appetite, energy stability, body composition, and long-term health often respond more strongly to food quality than to calorie arithmetic alone. Better food tends to reduce the need for constant management because it supplies what the body is actually asking for. It is richer in protein, steadier in fuel delivery, denser in regulatory nutrients, and more likely to finish the meal biologically. Lower-quality food often forces the eater into repeated negotiation with hunger, cravings, unstable energy, and compensatory eating because the body received heat without enough useful material. Abstract calorie totals miss this because they treat all incoming energy as if it were metabolically interchangeable. It is not. The body cares what the calories are made of, what they arrived with, what they displaced, and what remains after digestion is complete. That is why food quality matters more. It is closer to what the organism is actually measuring.

Reframing Diet as Inputs, Not Restrictions

Most people are taught to think about diet from the outside in. The central question becomes what to remove, what to avoid, what to limit, what rule to follow, what indulgence to resist, what number to stay under. That frame sounds disciplined, but it begins in the wrong place. The body does not experience a diet as a restriction plan. It experiences a stream of inputs. Every meal delivers or fails to deliver amino acids, fatty acids, glucose, minerals, vitamins, water, osmotic load, fiber bulk, plant defense chemistry, and hormonal instructions. The organism then has to process those inputs through stomach acid, bile flow, pancreatic enzymes, intestinal transport, liver sorting, cellular uptake, mitochondrial oxidation, tissue repair, and renal clearance. Once food is seen that way, diet stops looking like a moral struggle against appetite and starts looking like a problem of biological supply. The real issue is not how heroically a person can restrict himself. The real issue is what the body is being given to work with.

Restriction-based thinking hides the central nutritional failure point because it treats less food as inherently better food. But eating less of the wrong inputs does not solve the deeper problem if the remaining food still underdelivers protein, weakens satiety, destabilizes blood glucose, or leaves the body short on usable fats and regulatory nutrients. A person can follow a restrictive plan perfectly and still feed the organism badly. He can shrink calorie intake while keeping structural nutrition low. He can remove visible excess while preserving hidden deficiency. In that state, hunger becomes louder, energy more volatile, mood less stable, and adherence progressively harder. The usual interpretation is that the person lacks discipline. A more honest interpretation is that the body has been placed under a lower-input regime without receiving better inputs. The appetite system is then blamed for protesting an arrangement that never actually fed the organism properly.

An input-based frame asks a different set of questions. Did this meal deliver enough complete protein to support tissue repair, enzyme turnover, immune function, and stable satiety. Did it contain fats that can support membrane integrity, hormone synthesis, bile-responsive digestion, and longer fuel access. Did it provide minerals and vitamins in forms the intestine can absorb and the cell can use. Did it create a manageable glucose response or did it flood the bloodstream with rapid carbohydrate energy and force the pancreas into hard containment. Did digestion liberate meaningful nutrition, or did the food arrive with structural barriers, binding compounds, and low net yield. These questions sound more technical because they are closer to what the body is actually solving after every meal. They move the conversation away from permission and punishment and back toward supply, handling, and tissue consequence.

This shift changes the emotional tone of nutrition because it removes the false heroism of deprivation. The goal is no longer to win by enduring hunger, white-knuckling cravings, and obeying external rules with maximum purity. The goal is to build meals that reduce the biological reason for those problems to exist. When the body receives dense protein, useful fats, and stronger micronutrient support, appetite often becomes quieter because the meal resolves more of the organism's real demand. When meals are built around refined starch, sugar, and low-structure convenience foods, the body may be overexposed to energy while still underfed where it counts. In that state, the person is told to cut back. But the smarter move is often to improve the incoming material first. Better input changes the downstream equation more effectively than stricter restriction layered on top of poor food.

Reframing diet as inputs does not mean intake never matters. It means intake has to be interpreted through biological value. The body is not a storage bin that merely needs less stuff thrown into it. It is a living structure that must be rebuilt continuously while managing incoming fuel, stress, waste, and repair. A good diet therefore begins by supplying what the organism most needs and reducing what distorts that supply. Once that becomes the standard, the question stops being how little can I get away with eating. The question becomes what pattern of inputs leaves the body better built, more stable, less hungry, and less burdened after digestion is over. That is a much harder question than restriction. It is also the one that actually matters.

Chapter 5

The Industrial Food Environment

Before industrialization, food was still tied to the biological realities that produced it. Animals had to be raised, hunted, trapped, or fished. Fat had to be rendered from real tissue. Milk had to come from an actual animal in lactation. Eggs had to be laid. Plant foods had to be gathered in season, cultivated with labor, or preserved with methods that did not erase their original structure. This imposed hard limits on what could be eaten and in what form. A person could not casually surround himself with endless shelves of refined starch, extracted oils, sweetened drinks, and engineered snack products because those things did not yet exist at meaningful scale. Most food arrived with friction built into it. It spoiled. It required work. It carried the signature of the organism or plant it came from. Meat was still muscle, connective tissue, fat, blood, and organ matter. Dairy was still a fresh or fermented animal food, not a flavored chemical system. Grain, where it existed, was closer to an agricultural raw material than to the stabilized, fractionated powders that would later dominate industrial food manufacturing. The body was still meeting food in forms that resembled life, not factory design.

That matters because pre-industrial eating forced a closer relationship between nourishment and structure. Animal foods carried dense packages of complete protein, fat, minerals, and fat-soluble vitamins in forms digestion could access with relatively high efficiency. A piece of meat did not need to be reconstructed into usefulness by fortification. Its proteins could be denatured by gastric acid, cut into peptides and amino acids, absorbed, and put back into circulation as structural material. Its fats could be emulsified by bile, hydrolyzed by lipase, and used as stable fuel or membrane substrate. Organs concentrated vitamins, iron, copper, and other regulatory nutrients in tissues that made biological sense because those nutrients were already functioning in the animal they came from. Even when plant foods were eaten regularly, they existed inside a different hierarchy than they do now. They were often seasonal, more fibrous, less sweet, more variable, and far less chemically isolated. They accompanied life. They did not define the food system.

Pre-industrial diets also contained physical limits that modern people rarely account for when they talk about traditional eating patterns. Sugar was not everywhere because extracting and refining it at large scale was difficult and expensive. Seed oils were not standard household fats because taking a small amount of oil out of hard industrial seeds required mechanical force and chemical processing that most people did not have. Grain products were constrained by milling, spoilage, storage, and labor. Freshly milled flour still contained unstable components that shortened shelf life. Animal fat, by contrast, could be collected directly from the food animal, rendered, stored, and used as both cooking medium and energy source. This meant that the baseline food environment was biased toward foods that either came directly from animal tissue or remained closer to their natural agricultural form. The body was not being asked to manage a daily assault of hyper-palatable mixtures built from refined starch, concentrated sugar, extracted oils, stabilizers, emulsifiers, and flavor systems designed to override satiety. It was being fed inside narrower ecological and technological limits.

This does not mean every pre-industrial diet was ideal, nor does it mean all historical populations ate the same way. Geography, climate, animal access, season, class, and local agriculture all shaped what people lived on. But across that diversity, one feature remained more common than it is now. Food still had to answer to reality. It had to come from somewhere visible. It had to retain enough structural honesty that the eater could still recognize what organism or raw material it came from. That kept the conversation closer to biology even when no one used biochemical language. People were still eating food that behaved like food in the digestive tract, not edible products engineered for shelf life, repeat purchase, and sensory manipulation. Industrialization changed that relationship. It did not simply increase abundance. It inserted a manufacturing layer between the organism and the eater, and from that point forward the body increasingly had to process inventions rather than foods.

Refined Flour, Sugar, and Industrial Oils

Refined flour, sugar, and industrial oils form the biochemical base of the modern processed food system because they solve the manufacturer's problem while creating a very different problem for the body. They are cheap to produce at scale, easy to store, easy to transport, easy to standardize, and easy to combine into products that taste more intense than the raw agricultural materials they came from. But the processes that make them commercially useful are the same processes that strip them out of their original food context and change the way the body has to handle them. Grain becomes starch-heavy powder with much of its original structure removed. Sugar becomes concentrated sweetness without the physical limitations that once restrained intake. Seeds that would never have yielded large household amounts of oil through ordinary food preparation become major fat sources only after crushing, solvent extraction, refining, bleaching, and deodorizing. Each of these inputs is a simplification of a living material into a more industrially obedient ingredient. The factory gains control. The organism loses context.

Refined flour is what remains when grain is milled to last longer, feel softer, and behave predictably in manufacturing, even as more of the grain's original structure is stripped away. The fibrous outer layers and germ are removed, leaving a starch-dominant powder that stores more easily because much of the grain's unstable natural fat leaves with those discarded fractions. What enters the body is therefore not an intact seed structure but a concentrated carbohydrate substrate with much less physical resistance built into it. Once mixed, cooked, and eaten, refined flour products tend to break down quickly, generating glucose with relative ease compared with less processed plant structures. Protein quality remains poor relative to animal foods, mineral value is weakened further by grain chemistry and processing losses, and satiety is usually weaker than foods built around dense protein and natural fat. The product is easy to eat, easy to overeat, and metabolically thin relative to the status staple carbohydrates have been given.

Refined sugar intensifies that problem by removing even the minimal structural friction still present in flour. It enters the diet as concentrated sweetness with almost no structural value attached to it. No meaningful protein. No meaningful fat. Little to no micronutrient contribution in its refined form. What it delivers is fast carbohydrate energy and strong sensory reward. Once digested and absorbed, glucose and fructose handling begin quickly. Glucose raises blood sugar and drives insulin release. Fructose is handled heavily by the liver, where it can contribute to glycogen repletion, de novo lipogenesis, meaning new fat production, and a broader hepatic workload when intake is high and repeated. Sugar's metabolic problem is not simply that it contains calories. The problem is that it delivers rapidly accessible energy with weak structural payoff and a reward profile that can keep intake rising long after real nutritional needs were met. It satisfies the tongue faster than it satisfies the organism. That gap is part of why sugar-rich foods and drinks can leave appetite unstable. The body received fuel. It did not receive much construction material.

Industrial oils complete the triad by supplying an energy-dense fat source that exists at population scale only because of industrial processing. Seeds such as soybean, corn, cottonseed, sunflower, safflower, and canola do not yield large practical amounts of oil through ordinary kitchen methods. Their oils become major dietary fats only after intensive extraction and refining. The resulting products are uniform, shelf-stable, and useful for frying, emulsification, and processed food manufacturing. But from the body's perspective, this means a historically unusual volume of isolated polyunsaturated fatty acids is entering the diet in a form disconnected from the original seed matrix and often paired with refined flour and sugar in the same products. These oils are not arriving as part of an intact food that also supplies complete protein, robust micronutrient density, or strong satiety. They are often functioning as a cheap energy extender and texture enhancer inside foods already designed for repeated intake. Once absorbed, their fatty acids enter membrane systems, storage pools, and signaling pathways. That matters because membrane composition and inflammatory signaling are influenced by the types of fats the body is repeatedly asked to incorporate. The question is not whether a single dose of seed oil is a toxic event. The question is what kind of lipid environment repeated industrial oil exposure helps create over time when it displaces more stable and nutritionally coherent fats.

Together these three ingredients changed the food environment by separating energy from nourishment and speed from restraint. Refined flour supplies quickly accessible starch. Sugar supplies concentrated sweetness and rapid carbohydrate load. Industrial oils supply cheap dense fat that scales easily through manufacturing. Combine them and the result is food that is soft, shelf-stable, highly palatable, easy to chew, easy to swallow, and often weak in complete protein, weak in micronutrient density, and weak in durable satiety. The body can certainly process these ingredients to varying degrees. That is not the same as saying they fit human nutritional needs well when they become the base of the diet. A system built from tissue, enzymes, membranes, hormones, and mineral-dependent metabolism does not thrive on ingredients designed first for storage, profit, and sensory manipulation. Refined flour, sugar, and industrial oils did not merely add new options to the menu. They rewired the industrial diet around cheap fuel and low-friction intake, and the body has been paying for that redesign ever since.

Hyper-Palatable Food Engineering

Hyper-palatable food is not ordinary food that happens to taste good. It is food deliberately assembled to override normal stopping signals. The engineering begins with a simple industrial goal: make the product easy to chew, easy to swallow, highly rewarding on first contact, and weak in the kinds of friction that would normally slow intake. Real food usually carries some braking force. Meat requires chewing and produces strong satiety once protein digestion begins. Whole fruit contains water, fiber, bulk, and a finite sweetness locked inside plant structure. Eggs, dairy, tubers, and minimally processed starches still retain enough physical form that digestion unfolds at a more natural pace. Hyper-palatable food is different because the structure is redesigned to reduce resistance and intensify reward. Refined flour supplies soft, rapidly digestible starch. Sugar supplies concentrated sweetness and fast sensory impact. Industrial oils supply dense energy and mouthfeel. Salt amplifies flavor and suppresses blandness. Flavor chemistry sharpens the signal further. The result is a product that enters the mouth already optimized for continued intake before the stomach, intestine, pancreas, liver, and satiety system have had time to answer back.

Texture is part of the engineering, not a minor aesthetic detail. Crunch that dissolves quickly, creaminess without real structural density, crisp coatings over soft interiors, melt-in-the-mouth starch-fat combinations, all of these designs change how the body experiences the food. A product that collapses easily in the mouth can deliver a large amount of energy with very little chewing time, very little digestive anticipation, and very little mechanical effort. That matters because chewing and oral exposure help pace eating and contribute to the early signaling that prepares digestion. When food is designed to vanish quickly while remaining highly stimulating, intake can run ahead of satiety. The eater keeps receiving reward while the deeper biological systems are still catching up. This is one reason chips, pastries, ice cream, sweetened cereals, fast food sandwiches, and many packaged snack foods behave the way they do. They are not merely tasty. They are friction-reduced delivery systems for starch, sugar, fat, and flavor.

The body then receives a metabolically disordered signal. Energy arrives fast, but structural value is often low relative to the reward intensity. Protein may be minimal or incomplete. Micronutrient density is usually weak unless nutrients are added back artificially, and even then the product remains built on a refined base. Glucose may rise quickly. Insulin may have to rise accordingly. Fat extends the sensory reward and raises the energy load further. Salt keeps the product appetizing even after the palate would normally fatigue. Flavor systems create the illusion of richness beyond what the food's biological value would justify. The brain receives a strong message of desirability while the rest of the organism receives a far weaker message of nutritional sufficiency. This is the central trick. The product stimulates wanting more effectively than it resolves needing less.

Hyper-palatable food therefore disrupts appetite at the level of sequence. Normally, eating slows as gastric distension rises, digestion begins, amino acids and fatty acids appear, and satiety hormones such as cholecystokinin and peptide YY begin to signal that meaningful nourishment has arrived. When food is engineered to be rapidly consumable, intensely flavorful, and structurally thin, the reward curve can outrun the satiety curve. The person keeps eating into a lag. By the time the body starts fully responding, a large amount of energy has already entered. This is often described as poor self-control, but that explanation is shallow. The product was designed to create exactly this mismatch between sensory reward and biological completion. The eater is not weak because the food is pleasurable. The food is profitable because it was designed to keep pleasure high while stopping power stays delayed.

This is why hyper-palatable food engineering matters so much in the modern diet. It does not merely make food enjoyable. It changes the relationship between reward, satiety, and intake. It teaches the appetite system to live in an environment where taste intensity, softness, speed, and repeatability are artificially high while structural nutrition is often mediocre. Under those conditions, the body can become overfed in energy and underfed in real substance at the same time. The mouth is impressed. The tissues remain partly unconvinced. That gap is where repeated eating lives.

The Supermarket as a Metabolic Trap

The modern supermarket looks like abundance because it offers endless variation, but most of that variation sits on top of the same industrial base. Different brands, different colors, different textures, different health claims, but underneath the packaging the recurring structure is familiar: refined flour, refined sugar, industrial oils, flavor systems, emulsifiers, stabilizers, and synthetic fortification. The visual impression is diversity. The metabolic reality is repetition. The body is not walking into a neutral environment full of equally valid foods. It is being pushed into a retail system built to normalize products that deliver energy more reliably than they deliver structural nourishment. That is what makes the supermarket a metabolic trap. It teaches people to experience industrial food as ordinary food.

The layout reinforces the distortion. Real food is usually pushed to the edges: meat, eggs, dairy, some produce, sometimes seafood. The center aisles hold the real volume of branded choice, and that choice is dominated by shelf-stable products designed for storage, transport, and repeat purchase. Cereals, crackers, breads, bars, chips, frozen meals, desserts, sauces, sweetened drinks, snack foods, protein products that barely function as food once the marketing is stripped away. The structure of the store quietly teaches the shopper that packaged industrial products are the dietary center and that actual food is only one category among many. From the body's point of view, this means the default purchasing path is weighted toward foods that digest quickly, reward strongly, and often leave appetite unresolved. The trap is not merely that these products exist. The trap is that they have been made to feel foundational.

Packaging then adds another layer of deception by replacing physiology with language. A product does not need to feed the body well if it can signal virtue effectively. Low fat. Whole grain. Heart healthy. Organic. Plant based. High protein. Gluten free. Made with real fruit. Fortified with vitamins. These phrases do not explain what digestion will actually release from the product, what will remain bioavailable in the gut lumen, what kind of glucose and insulin response it is likely to produce, or whether it supplies enough complete protein, usable fat, and regulatory nutrients to support real satiety and tissue maintenance. They insert a narrative layer between the food and the organism. The shopper buys through claims. The body still has to process the underlying chemistry. This is how metabolically weak products are repeatedly sold under the visual language of responsibility.

Convenience makes the trap even stronger because convenience changes which foods win the decision before hunger has even been satisfied. Foods that require cooking, chewing, cleanup, refrigeration, and a little patience lose ground to foods that can be opened, poured, microwaved, or eaten while driving. But industrial convenience usually means structural simplification. More refinement. More fractionation. More soft starch. More concentrated sweetness. More isolated fat. More combinations engineered to move from hand to mouth with almost no resistance. That matters because resistance is part of normal eating. Chewing slows intake. Structure slows digestion. Whole food shape helps pace the meal. When food is softened, sweetened, flavored, and made instantly accessible, intake can rise long before the deeper satiety systems have time to answer. The shopper experiences this as ease. The organism experiences it as repeated metabolic pressure.

Price adds another layer because the cheapest food is often cheap for a physiological reason. It is built from subsidized commodity inputs that can be milled, extracted, flavored, colored, and stabilized into highly profitable products. The consumer feels he is saving money. The body is often paying with weaker protein intake, poorer fat quality, lower micronutrient density, weaker satiety, and more unstable energy regulation. Real nourishment usually costs more because actual animal foods, intact dairy, eggs, and other nutrient-dense foods are biologically more complex and less industrially obedient than flavored starch and extracted oils. Cheap processed food therefore does not simply offer low price. It offers a specific trade. Lower immediate cost in exchange for lower structural value and higher likelihood of repeated eating.

This is why the supermarket has to be read biologically rather than visually. The important distinction is not between branded categories, marketing stories, or the emotional tone of the packaging. It is simpler and harder than that. Which foods are still close to their original biological form. Which foods are mainly industrial assemblies disguised as nourishment. Once that line becomes visible, the store changes. It still contains traps, but they no longer look like normal food.

Why Cheap Calories and Real Nutrition Are Not the Same Thing

Cheap calories are cheap because they are easy to manufacture, easy to store, easy to transport, and easy to assemble into products that survive long supply chains. Real nutrition is more demanding. It has to arrive in forms the body can actually use. That difference is the whole problem. A calorie is only a unit of potential energy. It says nothing about whether the food delivering that energy also supplies complete amino acids, usable fats, bioavailable minerals, fat-soluble vitamins, or strong satiety signals. It says nothing about digestive burden, absorption efficiency, hormonal response, or net tissue value. A cheap food can flood the body with rapidly accessible fuel and still leave the organism structurally underfed. A more expensive food can deliver fewer total calories and yet provide far more of what the body actually needs to maintain muscle, enzymes, membranes, hormone production, immune function, and stable appetite. The price of the food and the biological value of the food are related only loosely. Industrial food economics rewards calorie production. Human physiology rewards usable nourishment.

This becomes clearer once food is judged by yield instead of volume. Refined starch, sugar, and industrial oils are cheap because they can be produced from large commodity streams and turned into shelf-stable ingredients with predictable behavior. They solve manufacturing problems beautifully. They do not solve human nutritional needs with the same elegance. Refined starch is easy to digest into glucose, but that does not make it rich in structural value. Sugar delivers quick carbohydrate energy, but almost no meaningful protein, almost no useful fat, and little micronutrient support in its refined form. Industrial oils add dense energy and mouthfeel, but they are often paired with weak protein content and weak overall nutrient density, especially inside processed foods. These ingredients can create fullness by volume or energy load for a moment, yet still leave the body looking for amino acids, minerals, and more durable satiety. The eater feels fed briefly. The organism remains partly unfinished.

Real nutrition behaves differently because it has to survive the full sequence from digestion to tissue use. A food is not valuable because it contains something on paper. It is valuable because digestion can release that material, the intestine can absorb it, the blood can carry it, and the tissues can use it without excessive waste or interference. Animal foods often perform well here because their proteins are complete, their fats are directly useful, and many of their vitamins and minerals arrive in forms the body can access with relatively high efficiency. Eggs, meat, dairy, and similar foods are not merely calorie sources. They are packages of construction material. The body can denature the proteins, absorb the amino acids, emulsify the fats, incorporate the lipids into membranes, and use the incoming nutrients to support repair and regulation. That is what real nourishment looks like. It is not abstract. It is material that survives contact with the digestive system and enters the organism in useful form.

Cheap calories also tend to distort appetite because they solve the least important part of hunger first. They solve the immediate energy gap. They do not necessarily solve the structural gap. A processed food can deliver a large amount of carbohydrate and fat very quickly, creating a strong reward signal and a fast rise in available energy. But if the same food is weak in complete protein, weak in micronutrient density, and weak in durable satiety, hunger returns because the body has not actually received enough of what it was asking for. This is why people can overeat low-cost processed food and still feel strangely unsatisfied. They are not always eating because they failed at self-control. Very often they are eating because the body keeps receiving disposable energy instead of full nourishment. Cheap calories keep the system running for the moment. Real nutrition helps finish the meal biologically.

This is why the supermarket and the modern food economy create such a deep illusion. The cheapest products often appear to be efficient because they deliver a lot of calories for very little money. But the body does not measure value that way. It measures what crossed the membrane, what stabilized energy, what supported repair, what reduced the need to keep eating, and what remained after digestion and clearance were complete. Cheap calories can be plentiful while real nutrition remains scarce. That is not a contradiction. It is one of the defining features of the industrial diet.

Part II

Human Digestive Design

Chapter 6

What Facultative Carnivore Means

The word omnivore sounds informative, but biologically it tells you very little. It only tells you that an organism can consume both plant and animal matter. It does not tell you what that organism is built to digest most efficiently, what foods supply its essential nutrients most directly, what kind of digestive architecture it carries, what fuel systems dominate under stable conditions, or how much biological work is required to turn one class of food into usable tissue compared with another. In other words, omnivore describes possibility, not priority. It describes range, not hierarchy. A species can be called omnivorous and still lean strongly toward one side of the food environment in terms of digestive compatibility, nutrient dependence, and metabolic design. That is the problem with using omnivore as if it settles the human food question. It does not settle anything. It only says that humans can eat more than one category of food without immediately dying.

That looseness matters because nutritional arguments are often built on the label as if it carries more precision than it actually does. Humans are omnivores, therefore grains are natural staples. Humans are omnivores, therefore plants and animals are nutritionally interchangeable so long as calories and a few nutrients are accounted for. Humans are omnivores, therefore any wide dietary pattern must be equally aligned with human biology as long as it keeps people alive. None of that follows from the word itself. An organism may tolerate a broad range of foods for survival reasons while still showing a clear physiological advantage when fed a narrower range of foods that better match its structure. Tolerance is not the same as optimization. Survival is not the same as design fit. The body's ability to endure a food is not proof that the food belongs at the center of the diet.

The digestive tract makes this visible. Humans do not possess the fermentation architecture of heavy plant-dependent animals. There is no rumen, no massive cecum, no digestive system built around prolonged microbial breakdown of cellulose as a primary means of energy extraction. The human stomach produces strong hydrochloric acid, a feature that aligns well with protein digestion and microbial defense in the handling of animal foods. The small intestine is the major site of absorption, and it is highly effective at taking up amino acids, fats, cholesterol, and other nutrients that animal foods supply densely. The colon can host fermentation, but it is not the dominant engine of human nourishment. This does not mean humans cannot eat plants. It means the word omnivore hides the fact that the human organism is not structurally organized like an animal that depends on plant bulk as its first nutritional principle.

The nutrient question sharpens the same point. Humans require complete amino acid input, highly usable fats, vitamin B12, bioavailable iron, zinc, and other nutrients that are supplied densely and directly by animal foods. Yes, the body can survive on mixed food strategies, use stored reserves, convert some compounds into others, and compensate for gaps through selective eating or supplementation. But that only proves flexibility. It does not prove equivalence. If one class of food delivers a larger share of essential nourishment in forms digestion can liberate and tissues can use with less interference, then calling the species omnivorous is descriptively true and still biologically incomplete. The label does not tell you where the nutritional center of gravity actually sits.

That is why the facultative carnivore framework is more precise. It keeps the flexibility that omnivore points to, but adds the missing hierarchy. Humans can eat a range of foods. That is the facultative part. But the underlying digestive and metabolic design still appears to favor dense animal-derived nutrition as the most direct route to structural repair, stable energy, and nutrient sufficiency. Omnivore leaves the reader with a broad permission slip. Facultative carnivore forces a more demanding question. Not what humans can eat, but what foods fit the organism best once digestion, absorption, tissue use, and long-term biological cost are taken seriously. That is the question the rest of this book is trying to answer.

Flexibility vs Preference in Biology

Biology often carries backup capacity, but backup capacity is not the same thing as design preference. A system can survive under multiple conditions while still functioning best under a narrower set of conditions. That distinction matters because people routinely confuse what an organism can tolerate with what the organism is built around. The human body can maintain blood glucose without dietary carbohydrate through gluconeogenesis, the endogenous production of glucose from amino acids, glycerol, and other substrates. It can also digest and use carbohydrate when carbohydrate is present. Both statements are true. But the coexistence of two capacities does not mean the body is expressing equal preference for both conditions. It means the body has options. In physiology, options are often survival tools. They protect the organism when food quality changes, seasons change, geography changes, or preferred inputs become scarce. Flexibility keeps the organism alive. Preference is revealed by what the anatomy, digestive sequence, nutrient dependencies, and metabolic pathways handle most directly and with the least compensatory work.

This principle appears everywhere in biology. A tissue can compensate for damage for a long time before failure becomes obvious. That compensation does not mean the damaged state is ideal. The kidney can preserve blood chemistry across wide conditions, but no one mistakes that reserve capacity for proof that all renal workloads are equally benign. The liver can detoxify a large range of compounds, but its ability to neutralize a burden does not convert that burden into nourishment. The same logic applies to food. Humans can eat mixed diets. Humans can survive on plant-heavy diets under some conditions. Humans can also shift toward heavier reliance on animal foods and maintain stable function there as well. The fact of flexibility is real. The mistake begins when flexibility is treated as a verdict that all dietary inputs are equally aligned with the organism. They are not. Some foods enter the digestive tract and yield dense, direct nourishment with relatively little obstruction. Others can be processed, but only after more binding, inhibition, fermentation, conversion, tolerance-testing, or clearing work. Survival capacity and preferred nutritional architecture are not the same biological event.

Preference is easier to see when you stop asking what can be swallowed and start asking what the body needs repeatedly. The human organism requires complete amino acids, membrane lipids, cholesterol-derived steroid substrates, bioavailable iron, vitamin B12, zinc, and a broad network of other nutrients that are delivered densely by animal foods. The stomach produces strong hydrochloric acid that denatures protein efficiently. The small intestine is highly effective at absorbing amino acids and fats. Bile physiology is built to manage lipid digestion. The colon can ferment some leftover material, but it is not built as a primary extraction chamber for fibrous plant bulk in the way heavy herbivorous systems are. This does not erase flexibility. It clarifies preference. The body can use other foods. The body is not built as though those foods are the central nutritional base.

Another way to see the difference is through cost. Preference usually reveals itself in the lower-friction path. Foods that supply nutrients in forms the body can access directly impose less digestive and metabolic negotiation. Animal foods generally deliver protein in complete form, fats in usable form, and minerals without the same degree of antinutrient binding that often complicates plant-based nutrition. Plant foods can still be eaten, sometimes successfully, but they are more variable. Their nutrient yield is often more dependent on preparation, quantity, host tolerance, and the presence or absence of compounds that interfere with digestion or absorption. A flexible organism can work around that. A preferred input does not require as much working around. That is the important difference. Preference is not about dogma. It is about where the system meets the least resistance while satisfying the greatest share of its recurring needs.

This is why the facultative carnivore frame matters. It keeps the flexibility without flattening the hierarchy. Humans are not obligate carnivores, but neither does their broad dietary tolerance prove that all foods occupy the same biological rank. The body carries fallback systems because life is unstable. That says something important about human adaptability. It does not erase the deeper question of which foods best fit the organism when the goal is not mere survival, but structural sufficiency, stable energy, and low-friction nourishment over time.

The Spectrum From Obligate Carnivory to Plant Dependence

Animals are often sorted into tidy dietary boxes, carnivore, omnivore, herbivore, as if those words were precise enough to settle real biological questions. They are not. The more honest view is a spectrum built from anatomy, digestive chemistry, nutrient dependence, and metabolic strategy. At one end are obligate carnivores, animals whose physiology is so tightly tied to animal tissue that survival depends on it. They require nutrients that are either absent from plant foods or unavailable in usable amounts unless they arrive already assembled inside another animal. Their digestive systems are built around protein and fat handling, their nutrient needs are centered on animal-derived material, and their metabolic flexibility in the plant direction is narrow. The term obligate matters because it means the organism is not merely advantaged by animal food. It is dependent on it. Remove that input and the system begins to fail.

Move away from that edge and the dependence softens, but the orientation can remain strongly animal-centered. Some species live as heavy carnivores without being absolute in the strictest sense. They may consume small amounts of non-animal material opportunistically, but the metabolic center of gravity remains animal tissue. Their digestion, dentition, stomach chemistry, and nutrient profile still point toward flesh, fat, and organ material as the dominant food environment. The occasional departure from that base does not redefine the design. It simply shows that life preserves fallback capacity when it can. This is the first place where confusion often begins. People see flexibility and assume equivalence. Biology does not make that leap. A system can deviate from its center without losing its center.

Further along the spectrum are species with broader adaptive range, the kinds of animals often compressed under the word omnivore. But even here the broad label hides hierarchy. Some animals classified as omnivores still lean strongly toward animal-derived nutrition because it supplies denser energy, more direct structural material, or more efficient nutrient capture relative to what their digestive architecture can do with plants. Others lean more heavily toward plant matter but retain the ability to exploit animal food when available. The important point is that omnivory is not a single biological condition. It is a wide middle zone containing very different organisms with very different priorities. One species may digest starch readily, another may rely much more on fat and protein, another may use plant foods often but still depend on occasional animal inputs for critical nutrients. The word itself tells you range. It does not tell you where on the range the organism actually lives best.

At the plant-dependent end of the spectrum, anatomy changes more dramatically because extracting meaningful nourishment from fibrous plant matter is hard work. Plant tissue stores much of its mass inside structural carbohydrate that vertebrate enzymes cannot digest directly. That forces the evolution of specialized fermentation systems. Large ceca, rumens, elongated digestive tracts, and microbial chambers become central because the animal is not primarily digesting plant structure itself. It is outsourcing that work to microbial populations capable of breaking cellulose and related compounds down into smaller molecules the host can then use. Plant dependence therefore demands architectural commitment. It is not just a preference for leaves over meat. It is a digestive redesign built around fermentation, prolonged retention time, microbial collaboration, and repeated recovery of fermentation products. A body built that way is telling you clearly what kind of food it depends on.

Humans become easier to place once the spectrum is viewed this way. They do not sit at the obligate carnivore end because they retain real flexibility and can use a variety of foods. But they also do not resemble plant-dependent animals in any serious structural sense. They do not carry a rumen. They do not carry a large fermentation apparatus capable of turning fibrous bulk into the dominant basis of nourishment. Their stomach acid is strong, their small intestine is central, their bile physiology is robust, and their nutrient requirements are met especially directly by animal foods that provide complete protein, usable fats, vitamin B12, bioavailable iron, zinc, and other critical compounds without the same degree of digestive obstruction or conversion burden found in many plant foods. This places humans somewhere inside the flexible middle, but not in a biologically neutral position. The spectrum matters because it shows that flexibility does not erase directional design. Humans may not be obligate carnivores, but neither are they built like animals whose nourishment depends primarily on plant fermentation. That narrower placement is exactly what the facultative carnivore framework is trying to name.

Why Humans Appear Metabolically Flexible but Structurally Animal-Food Oriented

Humans appear metabolically flexible because the body carries multiple fuel-handling pathways and can survive across a wide range of food environments. It can absorb carbohydrate and raise insulin in response to glucose. It can oxidize fat when carbohydrate intake falls. It can produce ketones from fatty acids and use them as a major fuel source, including in the brain. It can maintain blood glucose even in the absence of dietary carbohydrate through gluconeogenesis, the endogenous production of glucose from non-carbohydrate substrates such as amino acids and glycerol. That flexibility is real. It is one of the reasons humans have been able to spread across climates, seasons, and landscapes that offered very different food patterns. But flexibility in fuel handling is not the same thing as structural neutrality. The fact that the body can keep itself running under multiple dietary conditions does not mean all of those conditions nourish it equally well. A system can survive under pressure without revealing its preferred nutritional base.

The structural side of the question points more clearly toward animal foods. Human tissues are built from complete amino acid input, usable fats, cholesterol-derived steroid substrates, bioavailable minerals, and vitamins that are concentrated in animal foods with relatively little digestive obstruction. The body needs amino acids not only for muscle but for enzymes, transport proteins, immune molecules, gut lining turnover, connective tissue, and neurotransmitter synthesis. It needs fats not just as stored energy but as membrane material, signaling substrates, and carriers for fat-soluble vitamins. It needs vitamin B12, heme iron, zinc, preformed vitamin A in some contexts, creatine, carnosine, taurine, and other compounds that are either absent from plant foods, less concentrated in them, or require more conversion and more biological negotiation to obtain from them. Animal foods deliver these materials densely and in forms the digestive system can usually access directly. That matters because the organism is not built from dietary possibility. It is built from recurring material supply.

The digestive tract reflects the same orientation. Humans have a highly acidic stomach that denatures protein aggressively and creates a hostile environment for many foodborne microbes, a feature that makes sense in a species that can handle animal tissue regularly. The small intestine is the major site of nutrient extraction, and it is highly effective at absorbing amino acids, fats, cholesterol, and many minerals when they are presented in accessible form. Bile production and gallbladder release support fat digestion as a normal physiological event, not as an emergency detour. What humans do not have is the kind of fermentation-heavy digestive architecture seen in animals that depend primarily on fibrous plant bulk. There is no rumen, no large cecal system functioning as the main extraction chamber, no anatomy built around prolonged microbial conversion of cellulose into primary fuel. The colon can ferment leftovers. It does not define the diet. This means humans can process plant matter, but they are not structurally organized like animals whose nourishment depends on large-scale fermentation of plant fiber.

That is why the phrase metabolically flexible but structurally animal-food oriented matters. It separates fuel tolerance from nutritional center of gravity. A human can live on mixed diets, shift between glucose and fat use, tolerate seasonal carbohydrate, and survive under conditions that are far from ideal. But when the question changes from survival to biological fit, the answer narrows. The body's recurring structural needs are met more directly by foods that supply complete protein, usable fats, and densely bioavailable micronutrients with less interference and less conversion burden. Plant foods can still enter the picture. They may provide carbohydrate, variety, or context-dependent value. But the deeper architecture of the organism suggests that they function more as optional additions than as the core structural base. That is the distinction the facultative carnivore framework is trying to preserve. Humans are flexible enough to survive broadly. They still appear built to be nourished most directly by animal food.

What the Word "Facultative" Actually Clarifies

The word *facultative* clarifies the difference between capacity and design. Without it, the discussion collapses into a false binary. Either humans are treated as pure carnivores who cannot metabolize anything outside animal food, or they are treated as broad omnivores in a way that implies all major food classes are equally appropriate so long as they can be eaten and survived. *Facultative* breaks that mistake cleanly. It says the organism retains flexibility. It can function under more than one condition. But it also says that flexibility does not erase hierarchy. A body may carry fallback pathways, backup fuel systems, detoxification capacity, and broad dietary tolerance without being structurally indifferent to the foods it is given. That is what the word restores. It prevents survival range from being confused with nutritional center of gravity.

This matters because biology is full of facultative systems. A tissue can compensate before it fails. A cell can shift fuel use under changing conditions. An organism can tolerate environments that are not its best environment. None of those facts mean the alternatives are equal. They mean life protects itself with options. When applied to human nutrition, *facultative* says that humans can digest and metabolize a range of foods, including plant foods, starches, sugars, and mixed dietary patterns, but that this flexibility should not be mistaken for proof that those foods occupy the same biological rank as dense animal-derived nutrition. The stomach still has to denature protein. Bile still has to emulsify fat. The intestine still has to absorb usable amino acids, fats, vitamins, and minerals. The tissues still have to be built from what arrives. If one class of food supplies those recurring needs more directly, more densely, and with less obstruction, then flexibility does not flatten that advantage. It merely explains how the organism survives when that advantage is not fully available.

The word also clarifies why human nutrition has been so easy to misread. People often observe that humans can eat plants, grains, legumes, fruit, and tubers, then jump from that fact to a much larger conclusion that those foods must therefore be natural staples in the same foundational sense as animal foods. But *can use* is not the same as *best built around.* The body can run glucose metabolism. It can also run fat oxidation and ketone production. It can generate glucose internally through gluconeogenesis when dietary carbohydrate is absent. It can tolerate a wide range of food structures and chemical burdens to varying degrees. That broad tolerance is exactly why the word *facultative* is needed. It preserves the truth of adaptability without allowing adaptability to become a lazy argument for equivalence.

More specifically, *facultative* clarifies that the framework is not arguing for absolute exclusivity. It is not claiming that the mere presence of plant food is a biological emergency or that every non-animal food is equally harmful in every person under every condition. What it is saying is more precise. Animal foods appear to form the most direct structural base for human nourishment because they provide complete protein, usable fats, and a dense spectrum of bioavailable nutrients in forms that match human tissues and digestive priorities closely. Other foods may still be included. Some may be tolerated well. Some may serve context-dependent roles. Some may be harmless in modest amounts. But once the word *facultative* is understood, those foods stop being automatically treated as foundational. They are judged as optional inputs whose value depends on dose, preparation, host tolerance, metabolic condition, and what they displace.

That is the real usefulness of the term. It narrows the argument without making it brittle. It protects the framework from the simplistic charge that if humans can eat many things, then hierarchy must disappear. It also protects it from the opposite simplification that flexibility must be denied in order to make a serious case for animal-food centrality. *Facultative* says the body has range. It also says range is not the same as nutritional equality. That is the clarification the word brings, and without that clarification the entire discussion immediately becomes less exact.

Chapter 7

Human Digestive Anatomy

The digestive tract is not a passive tube that food falls through on its way to becoming energy. It is a staged processing system that decides, step by step, what from the outside world is allowed to become part of the body. That distinction matters because food is not internal the moment it is swallowed. Until digestion breaks it down, until the intestinal lining permits absorption, until nutrients cross a membrane and enter circulation, the contents of the digestive tract are still physically outside the organism in an important biological sense. The gut lumen, the hollow interior space of the digestive tract, is not yet the bloodstream, not yet the liver, not yet the cell. It is a controlled exposure chamber. Food enters that chamber as foreign material made of proteins, fats, carbohydrates, minerals, water, microbes, plant defense chemicals, connective tissue, cellulose, starch granules, and countless other structures the body cannot use in their original form. The job of the digestive tract is to reduce, sort, dismantle, and filter that material until usable fractions can be admitted and unusable or dangerous fractions can be contained and eliminated.

That work begins mechanically. Teeth break food into smaller particles. The tongue positions it. Saliva wets it and begins limited chemical processing. Swallowing then moves the food bolus into the stomach, where the environment changes sharply. Hydrochloric acid lowers pH, denatures proteins, alters microbial survival, and activates pepsin so large protein structures can start coming apart. The stomach also churns. It does not simply store. It grinds, mixes, liquefies, and meters. This is important because digestion is partly a problem of surface area and timing. Large intact structures are hard for enzymes to access. Smaller, acid-exposed, mechanically disrupted particles are easier to process. By the time food leaves the stomach, it is no longer a recognizable meal in the ordinary sense. It has been converted into chyme, a semi-liquid mixture that can be delivered in controlled amounts into the small intestine for deeper chemical handling.

The small intestine is the central extraction zone. Here, pancreatic enzymes cut proteins into peptides and amino acids, starches into absorbable sugars, and fats into smaller lipid fractions after bile acids have emulsified them into microscopic droplets. The intestine does not merely bathe food in enzymes and hope for the best. Its lining is built for contact and transfer. Folds, villi, and microvilli expand surface area dramatically so the absorptive membrane can do real work. Amino acids cross through transport proteins. Sugars move through dedicated carriers. Lipid digestion products are assembled into transport particles and routed into lymphatic circulation. Minerals and vitamins are absorbed with varying degrees of efficiency depending on chemical form, digestive conditions, and the presence of compounds that may bind or inhibit them. This is where many nutritional illusions collapse. A food may contain something valuable on paper, but if digestion cannot liberate it cleanly, if it remains bound in the lumen, if it is degraded before absorption, or if the transport conditions are poor, then the nutrient does not become nourishment in full biological terms. The food entered the tract. The body still did not receive the promised value.

Seen this way, the digestive tract is less like a pipe and more like an industrial sorting and refining line, except the material being processed is chemically active and the machinery is alive. Acid, enzymes, bile, mucus, peristalsis, transporters, barrier proteins, immune surveillance, microbial populations, and hormonal feedback all work together to decide what gets admitted, what gets delayed, what gets transformed, and what gets rejected. The liver then receives much of what is absorbed and performs another round of sorting, storage, conversion, and detoxification. The colon handles what remains, absorbing water, exposing leftover material to microbial fermentation, and compacting waste for elimination. At every stage the organism is making decisions. Use this. Break this down further. Keep this out. Clear this later. What looks from the outside like eating is, from the inside, a prolonged series of controlled processing events that determine whether food becomes tissue, fuel, burden, or waste.

This is why digestive anatomy matters so much in any serious discussion of human nutrition. Foods are not equal simply because they can be chewed and swallowed. They differ in how much force, acid, enzymatic work, bile handling, and absorptive precision they demand. They differ in what they yield after all that work is done. Some foods move through this system in a way that produces dense, usable nutrition with relatively little obstruction. Others arrive with more friction, more binding chemistry, more structural resistance, or more metabolic cleanup attached. The digestive tract is where those differences become real. It is the first place where dietary reputation collides with physiology, and physiology is the part that wins.

Mouth, Stomach, Small Intestine, Liver, Gallbladder, Pancreas, Colon

Digestion begins in the mouth, but not in the simplistic sense people usually mean when they say chewing is important. The mouth is the first mechanical reduction chamber, the first contact point between food and the body's processing system. Teeth fracture muscle fibers, crush softer tissues, and reduce plant matter into smaller particles so enzymes and acid can reach more surface area later. Saliva wets the bolus, lubricates swallowing, and begins limited carbohydrate digestion through salivary amylase, though that contribution is brief once food reaches the acid of the stomach. More important is the signaling function. Tasting, chewing, and swallowing begin the cephalic phase of digestion, the anticipatory response in which the nervous system prepares downstream organs for incoming food. Gastric acid secretion begins to rise. Pancreatic output is primed. The gut is told to get ready. A meal that passes through the mouth too quickly weakens part of that sequence. It reaches the stomach with less mechanical preparation and often with less coordinated digestive readiness.

The stomach is the first true chemical disassembly chamber. Its job is not simply to hold food but to acidify it, denature it, mix it, and meter it. Hydrochloric acid lowers the gastric pH enough to unfold proteins, turning tightly folded structures into exposed chains that proteases can actually cut. Pepsin begins the first major step of protein digestion. Connective tissue softens. Microbial burden is reduced. The stomach also churns aggressively, converting the swallowed meal into chyme, a semi-liquid mass that can be delivered into the small intestine in controlled pulses rather than dumped all at once. This pacing matters because the small intestine has to be able to neutralize acid, receive enzymes, emulsify fat, and absorb nutrients without being overwhelmed. The stomach is therefore not a bag. It is a regulated acid mixer that decides when the next stage can begin and in what form the meal will arrive.

The small intestine is where the real extraction happens. If the stomach begins the dismantling, the small intestine performs the fine work of turning food into absorbable fractions. Pancreatic enzymes enter here and cut proteins into smaller peptides and amino acids, carbohydrates into simple sugars, and fats into absorbable lipid fragments after bile has emulsified them. The lining is built for contact. Folds increase area. Villi project into the lumen. Microvilli cover the absorptive cells and create a dense brush border where final digestion and transport occur. This is not passive absorption. Specific transporters pull amino acids, glucose, minerals, and other molecules across the epithelial barrier. Lipid fragments are repackaged into chylomicrons and sent into lymphatic circulation because fat cannot simply dissolve into portal blood the way water-soluble nutrients can. This is also where many foods reveal their real value or lack of it. Nutrients that remain trapped, bound, insoluble, or chemically obstructed do not become nourishment merely because they were swallowed. The small intestine is where food has to prove it can actually cross into the body.

The liver sits just downstream as the first great sorting organ. Most absorbed nutrients coming from the small intestine enter the portal circulation and are delivered directly to the liver before they are allowed wider access to the body. That gives the liver enormous control. It stores glucose as glycogen or releases it depending on need. It converts amino acids, processes nitrogen into urea for later renal excretion, handles vitamins and minerals, assembles lipoproteins, and detoxifies compounds that should not circulate freely. The liver is also the site of bile production, linking it directly to fat digestion as well as metabolic sorting. This means the liver is both a digestive support organ and a metabolic command center. It decides what can be stored, what must be transformed, what gets released, and what needs to be neutralized. A diet that repeatedly sends unstable glucose surges, excess fructose burden, poorly handled fats, alcohol, or chemical waste through this system changes the liver's workload profoundly. Food is not simply absorbed. It is interrogated here.

The gallbladder is smaller, but its role is decisive when dietary fat arrives. Bile made by the liver is stored and concentrated in the gallbladder until it is needed. When fat reaches the duodenum, the hormone cholecystokinin signals the gallbladder to contract and release bile into the small intestine. Bile acids then act as detergents, surrounding fat droplets and breaking them into much smaller particles so pancreatic lipase can work on them. Without this step, large fat globules remain poorly accessible and absorption falls apart. The gallbladder therefore turns a steady trickle of liver-made bile into a timed surge matched to the meal. This is one reason the body handles a fat-rich meal very differently from a carbohydrate-rich one. Fat digestion requires coordinated release, emulsification, and transport. The system is built for it, but it is not casual.

The pancreas is the enzyme engine. It releases bicarbonate to neutralize gastric acid as chyme leaves the stomach, protecting the intestinal lining and creating the pH range in which digestive enzymes can function properly. It also secretes proteases for proteins, lipase for fats, and amylase for carbohydrates. That already makes it indispensable to digestion, but the pancreas also controls one of the central endocrine signals in metabolism through insulin and glucagon. This means the same organ that helps break down food also helps determine what the body does with the absorbed nutrients once they enter circulation. It sits at the bridge between digestion and metabolic regulation. Poor pancreatic function therefore affects both sides of the equation. Food may not be broken down effectively, and nutrient partitioning may become unstable even when breakdown occurs.

The colon, or large intestine, is the final handling zone. By the time food reaches it, most absorbable protein, fat, and simple carbohydrate should already be gone. What remains is water, electrolytes, microbial biomass, indigestible material, unabsorbed residues, bile-derived compounds, and whatever escaped earlier processing. The colon reclaims water and certain salts, compresses waste, and hosts dense microbial fermentation of leftover substrates. This fermentation can produce short-chain fatty acids from some fibers and resistant starches, along with gas and a wide range of metabolic byproducts. The colon is therefore not where most human nourishment is extracted, but it is where leftovers are negotiated. In a well-matched diet, that work remains limited and orderly. In a mismatched diet heavy in poorly digested or highly fermentable material, the colon becomes a site of bloating, excess gas, irritation, altered motility, and microbial disorder. What reaches the colon says something important about what earlier digestive stages did well and what they failed to finish.

Taken together, these organs form a continuous processing system rather than a collection of separate parts. The mouth prepares. The stomach acidifies and denatures. The small intestine extracts. The liver sorts. The gallbladder times bile delivery. The pancreas provides enzymatic force and metabolic regulation. The colon recovers water and handles residues. Food has to pass through all of them. That is why any serious discussion of nutrition has to start here. A diet is never just a set of ingredients. It is a repeated workload imposed on a living anatomical system.

Why Digestive Architecture Matters When Judging Food

A food cannot be judged honestly until it has been judged against the structure that has to process it. That is the first correction. Most nutrition language treats food as if value were obvious from the outside. A label lists protein, carbohydrate, fat, fiber, vitamins, minerals, and calories, and the public is taught to assume the body will receive those things more or less as advertised. But the body never encounters food in label form. It encounters physical matter entering a digestive machine with specific limits, strengths, and priorities. The stomach has to acidify it. The pancreas has to release the right enzymes against it. The liver and gallbladder have to support fat handling through bile production and release. The small intestine has to liberate the useful fractions and move them across a membrane without too much interference. The colon has to deal with what remains. Food is therefore not judged by what it contains in isolation. It is judged by what the digestive architecture can actually do with it. If the food arrives in a form that this architecture can dismantle cleanly and absorb efficiently, its value rises. If it arrives with more structural resistance, more binding chemistry, more fermentable residue, or more dependence on microbial salvage and host tolerance, its real value falls no matter how impressive it looked on paper.

This is why animal foods and many plant foods do not enter the body on equal terms. Animal tissue generally comes with proteins the stomach can denature and proteases can cut into complete amino acid pools with high efficiency. Its fats can be emulsified by bile and hydrolyzed by lipase into lipid fragments the intestine knows how to absorb. Many of its minerals arrive without the same degree of plant-associated binding chemistry that can reduce access in the gut lumen, the interior space where digestion and absorption are taking place. By contrast, many plant foods package their nutrients inside fibrous cell walls, starch structures, seed matrices, lectins, phytates, oxalates, tannins, or other defensive compounds that either slow access, reduce digestibility, or interfere directly with absorption. None of this means plant foods are indigestible in an absolute sense. It means they place different demands on the digestive tract and often deliver less usable nutrition relative to what they appear to contain. The same intestine that absorbs amino acids and fats from animal foods with relatively direct efficiency may have to negotiate far more chemistry to extract a smaller share of useful material from a seed, grain, or fibrous plant food.

Digestive architecture also matters because humans are not built like animals that rely on large-scale fermentation as the main route to nourishment. There is no rumen, no enormous cecal chamber, no digestive design centered on prolonged microbial breakdown of cellulose as a primary source of usable energy. The human system is organized around a strong acid stomach, a long and absorptively powerful small intestine, bile-dependent fat handling, and enzyme-driven digestion of proteins, fats, and more accessible carbohydrates. That architecture tells you what kinds of foods the body handles most directly. It is not neutral. It does not flatten all edible matter into nutritional equality. A food that depends heavily on fermentation to unlock value, or that sends a large volume of low-yield bulk into the colon, is not meeting this system where it is strongest. A food that arrives as dense protein, usable fat, and relatively accessible micronutrient material is.

This is why digestive architecture changes the standard of judgment completely. The real question is no longer whether a food belongs to a praised category or whether it contains fashionable nutrients. The real question is what the body has to spend in order to get value from it. How much acid. How much bile. How much enzymatic force. How much tolerance for antinutrients, irritants, or fermentable residue. How much cleanup later. A food that nourishes with less friction has a different biological status from a food that must be soaked, sprouted, fermented, pressure cooked, combined, fortified, and tolerated carefully before it can deliver a fraction of what another food supplies directly. The digestive tract is not a background detail in nutrition. It is the proving ground. A food's reputation enters the mouth. Its real value is decided by the organs that have to process it.

Why the Human System Is Not Built Like a Heavy Plant-Fermentation System

A heavy plant-fermentation system is built around one central problem: how to turn fibrous plant structure into usable nourishment when the animal itself cannot digest that structure directly. Plant cell walls contain cellulose and related carbohydrates that resist the digestive enzymes mammals normally secrete. To extract significant value from that material, the digestive tract has to outsource the work to microbes. That requires architecture. Large fermentation chambers, prolonged retention time, specialized gut compartments, enlarged ceca, which are pouch-like structures at the beginning of the large intestine, or rumens, the major fermentation chambers found in ruminants. These structures are not minor accessories. They are the core machinery of plant dependence. Food is held, softened, fermented, and reworked for long periods while microbial populations break down tough plant matter into smaller compounds the host can then absorb and use. A body built this way is telling you something clear. Its nourishment depends heavily on microbial conversion of fibrous bulk.

The human system is organized differently. The stomach is highly acidic. The small intestine is long, enzyme-driven, and central to nutrient extraction. Bile production and pancreatic enzyme release are robust, which matters especially for the digestion of protein and fat. The colon can ferment leftovers, but it is not the primary engine of human nourishment. By the time material reaches the large intestine, the major work of protein digestion, fat digestion, and much of carbohydrate absorption should already be finished. What remains is water recovery, microbial handling of residual material, and waste formation. That is a very different arrangement from a system that depends on large upstream fermentation chambers to unlock the majority of its calories and nutrients. Humans do have a microbiome. They do produce short-chain fatty acids from some fermentable fibers. But that contribution sits downstream and secondary. It does not define the digestive design.

This matters because many modern nutrition arguments speak as if humans were built to thrive on large amounts of fibrous plant bulk in the same way heavily fermenting herbivorous systems are. The anatomy does not support that assumption. A rumen animal can hold and ferment plant matter for extended periods because its digestive structure is built around that task. A large-cecum fermenter is still investing major anatomical real estate into microbial extraction. Humans are not doing that. They are relying far more on acid denaturation, enzymatic cleavage, membrane transport, and relatively direct absorption in the small intestine. That means foods which supply dense, accessible protein and fat meet the system closer to its strengths. Foods that depend heavily on fermentation, prolonged microbial breakdown, or tolerance for large amounts of indigestible bulk do not.

This is also why plant foods behave so variably in humans. Some are tolerated well in modest amounts. Some provide useful carbohydrate. Some create bloating, gas, altered transit, or irritation when dose rises or gut tolerance is poor. That variability is not mysterious. It reflects the fact that the human colon can do some salvage work, but the system is not built like a dedicated fermentation machine. When large amounts of fibrous, resistant, or chemically defended plant matter reach the lower gut, microbes will act on it. Gas, osmotic shifts, distension, and altered motility are common outputs of that interaction. In a true heavy plant-fermentation system, that microbial processing is the center of the design. In humans, it is more often a secondary negotiation with what earlier digestion did not or could not fully handle.

So the point is not that humans cannot eat plants. The point is that the digestive tract is giving away its priorities. Strong stomach acid, powerful small-intestinal absorption, bile-dependent fat handling, and the absence of a major fermentation apparatus all indicate a system that is not organized around turning fibrous plant mass into primary nourishment. The human body can ferment some leftovers. That is not the same as being built to live through fermentation as its main nutritional strategy.

Chapter 8

Digestive Differences Between Foods

Digestion does not begin when food reaches the stomach. It begins when the body decides that food is coming. Sight, smell, anticipation, chewing, and taste all feed into the cephalic phase of digestion, the early neurological stage in which the brain starts preparing the gut before the meal has fully arrived. Saliva rises. Gastric acid secretion begins to increase. The pancreas is primed. Bile handling is set into motion. Motility changes. This matters because the digestive tract is not a passive drainpipe waiting for material to drop through it. It is a responsive processing system that adjusts itself according to what kind of food it expects to handle. A protein-rich meal and a sweet drink do not ask the same thing of the body. One requires strong acid, proteolysis, which is enzymatic cutting of protein into smaller fragments, and slower downstream handling. The other may move rapidly, raise blood glucose quickly, and require much less mechanical and chemical dismantling before absorption begins. Digestion is therefore not simply breakdown. It is interpretation.

The stomach makes this visible. When food enters, the body is not only dealing with volume. It is reading composition. Protein triggers a strong gastric response because the proteins must be denatured by hydrochloric acid before enzymes such as pepsin can access them effectively. Fat slows gastric emptying and helps trigger cholecystokinin, a digestive hormone that signals bile release and pancreatic enzyme secretion. Refined carbohydrate behaves differently. It often exits the stomach more quickly, especially when fiber, protein, and fat are minimal, and moves into the small intestine where glucose can begin appearing in the bloodstream with relative speed. These are different digestive programs.

The same gut is being used, but it is being used under different instructions. Food is telling the system how urgently to acidify, how much bile to release, how aggressively to secrete enzymes, how fast to move the meal forward, and how quickly nutrients are likely to enter circulation. That is what it means to call digestion signal-driven. The meal is not just being acted upon. It is shaping the action.

This is one reason why mixed modern meals can create such metabolic confusion. A meal built from refined starch, sugar, industrial fat, flavor systems, and weak protein is not simply "food" in a neutral sense. It delivers competing instructions. Fast carbohydrate pushes toward rapid glucose absorption and insulin response. Fat slows emptying and extends exposure. Weak protein leaves structural demand partly unresolved. Hyper-palatable texture encourages intake before satiety has time to build. The result is a digestive event in which reward can outrun completion. The body receives a high-energy load, but the signals for tissue-building sufficiency and durable satiety are often weaker than the sensory intensity of the meal would suggest. This is why the same number of calories can behave so differently depending on food composition. The digestive tract is not processing an abstract energy total. It is responding to a set of chemical cues that determine timing, hormone release, fuel partitioning, and ultimately whether the meal feels finished or keeps pushing the eater toward more.

Once digestion is understood as a signal-driven system, food categories stop looking interchangeable. The important question is no longer simply what the food contains. The deeper question is what the food tells the body to do. Does it call for strong acid and protein breakdown because dense structural material has arrived. Does it call for bile and lipase because stable fat is entering the gut. Does it create a rapid glucose surge that forces immediate containment. Does it slow the meal down, increase satiety signaling, and deliver usable material over time, or does it move fast, reward hard, and leave the organism biologically underfinished. That is where digestive differences between foods become real. The gut is not merely breaking food apart. It is reading it, and then building a physiological response around what it sees.

Protein Digestion, Fat Digestion, Carbohydrate Digestion

Protein, fat, and carbohydrate do not enter the body as equivalent fuel units waiting to be tallied. They enter as different physical problems, and the digestive tract answers each one with a different sequence of chemistry, timing, and transport. Protein arrives as folded molecular structure. Before the body can use it, the stomach has to acidify the meal strongly enough to denature those proteins, meaning unfold them so their peptide bonds become accessible. Pepsin begins cutting them into smaller fragments, and then pancreatic proteases in the small intestine continue the work until amino acids and small peptides can cross the intestinal lining. Fat arrives as a different kind of challenge because it does not mix with the watery environment of the gut. The body cannot simply expose a large fat globule to enzymes and expect efficient access. Bile acids have to emulsify it first, breaking it into microscopic droplets that expand surface area. Pancreatic lipase then hydrolyzes triglycerides into fatty acids and monoglycerides, which are packaged for absorption and sent into lymphatic transport rather than directly into portal blood. Carbohydrate follows a faster path. Starches and sugars are reduced into absorbable sugars through salivary and pancreatic amylase and brush-border enzymes in the small intestine. Glucose can then move into circulation quickly, often producing a rapid endocrine response through insulin. These are not variations on the same digestive event. They are separate programs running through the same organs.

Protein digestion is the most obviously structural of the three because what is being extracted is not only energy potential but raw material the body uses to build itself. That is why stomach acid matters so much. Without adequate acid, proteins are not denatured efficiently, pepsin is not activated well, and larger fragments can move forward before the meal has been properly prepared. Once those proteins reach the small intestine, the pancreas takes over with trypsin, chymotrypsin, and related enzymes that reduce peptide chains further, and the brush border completes the final trimming into absorbable units. The result is an amino acid supply that can be used for muscle maintenance, enzyme turnover, immune signaling, connective tissue repair, and a wide range of other structural needs. Protein digestion is therefore slower and more demanding than simple sugar handling, but it yields something fundamentally different. It feeds the organism at the level of construction.

Fat digestion is slower for a different reason. The issue is not folding and denaturation, but hydrophobicity, the tendency of fat to separate from water. The digestive system solves this by treating fat like an emulsification problem before treating it like an enzyme problem. The liver makes bile, the gallbladder stores and concentrates it, and when fat reaches the duodenum the body releases that bile into the lumen so fat droplets can be dispersed into a form pancreatic lipase can actually act on. After hydrolysis, the resulting lipid fragments are assembled into micelles, absorbed by intestinal cells, reassembled into triglycerides, and packaged into chylomicrons for lymphatic delivery. That long route matters because it helps explain why dietary fat usually produces a slower and steadier post-meal energy pattern. It is not simply absorbed and dumped into immediate glucose-like handling. It moves through a more elaborate digestive and transport sequence, one that also carries fat-soluble vitamins and contributes strongly to satiety by slowing gastric emptying and extending nutrient delivery over time.

Carbohydrate digestion is usually the fastest and least mechanically resistant of the three, especially when the carbohydrate is refined. Starch structures are broken down quickly, sugars often require little dismantling at all, and the resulting glucose can appear in portal blood with relatively little delay compared with the digestive labor required for protein and fat. That speed is exactly why carbohydrate behaves differently metabolically. A fast substrate enters circulation, pancreatic insulin rises, tissues take up glucose, glycogen may be replenished, and excess energy may be pushed toward storage if immediate demand is limited. In whole-food form, where carbohydrate remains embedded in tougher structure and arrives alongside fiber, water, protein, or fat, the pace can be moderated. In refined form, much of that resistance is gone. Carbohydrate then behaves less like a sustained nutritional package and more like a fast fuel signal. That is useful in some contexts and destabilizing in others. The body can certainly handle it. The point is that it handles it through a very different program from the one used for protein and fat.

This is why it is misleading to talk about food as if all macronutrients are interchangeable once swallowed. Protein digestion is about structural extraction. Fat digestion is about emulsification, lipid transport, and sustained fuel access. Carbohydrate digestion is about fast sugar delivery and its endocrine consequences. The digestive tract knows these differences even when nutrition culture pretends not to. It responds to each macronutrient with different secretions, different timing, different transport routes, and different downstream signaling. That is where the real distinction between foods begins.

Why Different Foods Trigger Different Digestive Programs

Different foods trigger different digestive programs because the body is not reacting to a generic object called food. It is reacting to chemistry, structure, and the kind of work required to make that chemistry usable. A steak, an egg, a potato, a bowl of berries, a spoonful of sugar, and a pastry made from refined flour and industrial oil do not present the same problem to the digestive tract. One arrives as dense animal protein wrapped in connective tissue and fat. Another arrives as starch locked inside plant structure. Another arrives already close to absorbable sugar. Another arrives as a soft industrial mixture engineered to move through the mouth quickly and flood the body with rapidly available energy. The body has to read those differences immediately because digestion is costly. Acid production, bile release, pancreatic enzyme secretion, gut motility, hormonal signaling, and membrane transport all consume resources. The organism cannot process every meal as if it were chemically identical. It has to select the right program for what just entered.

Protein-rich food tends to trigger one of the strongest digestive responses because protein is structurally complex and must be dismantled carefully. The stomach raises hydrochloric acid output to denature protein, meaning unfold its structure so enzymes can reach the peptide bonds holding amino acids together. Pepsin begins cutting those chains, and later pancreatic proteases continue the work in the small intestine. A meal rich in protein also tends to slow gastric emptying and stimulate satiety hormones because the body interprets the arrival of amino acids as a serious nutritional event. Structural material is coming in. Digestion needs time. Extraction needs to be efficient. This is a very different program from the handling of a sweet drink or refined carbohydrate snack, where the digestive tract can move quickly because less dismantling is needed before glucose begins appearing in circulation.

Fat triggers a different program because fat is not soluble in the watery environment of the gut. The body cannot simply pour enzymes onto a large fat globule and expect good access. It has to bring in bile from the liver and gallbladder to emulsify the fat into tiny droplets, increasing surface area so pancreatic lipase can work. This process changes timing. Fat slows gastric emptying, extends digestive contact, stimulates cholecystokinin, and creates a longer, steadier nutrient delivery profile. That slower pattern is not accidental. It reflects the fact that lipid handling is a more elaborate logistical problem than fast sugar absorption. The body is not merely receiving calories from fat. It is managing a hydrophobic substance that must be emulsified, hydrolyzed, repackaged, and transported through lymph before entering wider circulation.

Carbohydrate, especially refined carbohydrate, triggers yet another program because much of the digestive work is easier and faster. Starches can be broken down by amylases. Sugars may require very little dismantling at all before absorption. Once glucose enters the bloodstream, insulin signaling rises to contain and distribute it. The speed of this sequence is exactly why carbohydrate-rich foods can feel different in the body. When the carbohydrate is embedded in more intact structure, paired with protein and fat, or slowed by tougher food architecture, the glucose rise may be more controlled. When the carbohydrate is refined, softened, sweetened, and stripped of structural resistance, the entire event accelerates. The body shifts into rapid fuel management rather than prolonged extraction. That is a different digestive program because it is solving a different problem.

This is also why mixed modern foods can be so disruptive. A processed food built from refined starch, sugar, industrial fat, salt, and flavor chemistry forces several digestive signals to fire at once in an unbalanced way. Sugar pushes toward rapid absorption. Fat slows emptying. Weak protein means little structural completion. Hyper-palatable texture encourages continued eating before the deeper satiety systems have caught up. The body is then trying to run multiple digestive instructions on a food that was engineered for sensory reward rather than biological coherence. That mismatch is part of why some foods feel hard to stop eating and why others create bloating, unstable energy, or a quick return of hunger even when the calorie load was substantial.

So different foods trigger different digestive programs because they are different physical and chemical events. The body reads protein as a structural extraction problem, fat as an emulsification and transport problem, and carbohydrate as a speed-of-fuel problem. Food quality, refinement, and composition then determine how cleanly or chaotically those programs run. The digestive tract is not applying one universal script. It is selecting from several, and the kind of food placed into the system determines which one takes over.

Why Mixed Modern Meals Often Create Conflicting Digestive Signals

Mixed modern meals often create conflicting digestive signals because they combine ingredients that push the body in opposite directions at the same time. A meal built from refined starch, sugar, industrial fat, weak protein, flavor chemistry, and soft texture does not arrive as one coherent nutritional message. It arrives as a cluster of competing instructions. Fast carbohydrate says move quickly, absorb glucose, raise insulin, and manage immediate fuel. Fat says slow gastric emptying, release bile, extend digestion, and lengthen absorption. Protein, when present only in token amounts, is often too weak to create the strong satiety and structural signaling that a truly protein-rich meal would produce. The digestive system is then forced to run multiple programs on a product that was not designed for physiological clarity. It was designed for taste, convenience, and repeat intake. That is the first problem. The meal is sensory-coherent and metabolically incoherent.

A simple animal-based meal usually gives the body a clearer sequence. Protein and fat arrive together in forms the system is built to process. Gastric acid rises. Protein denatures. Pepsin begins cutting. Bile release is coordinated with fat entry into the small intestine. Pancreatic enzymes continue the breakdown. Satiety builds as amino acids and fatty acids begin to appear in circulation. The signals reinforce each other. A modern mixed meal often does the opposite. Refined carbohydrate wants rapid exit from the stomach and fast glucose entry into the bloodstream. Fat slows that movement down. Sweetness and flavor intensity drive continued eating before gastric fullness and hormonal satiety have fully registered. The mouth receives a strong reward signal while the gut receives a confusing workload. The body is trying to contain fast energy, digest fat, manage osmotic load, and figure out whether any meaningful structural material has actually arrived. That is not one message. It is a metabolic argument.

This conflict matters because digestion is timed. The stomach, pancreas, liver, gallbladder, intestine, and endocrine system are constantly trying to match secretions and transport to the food in front of them. When a meal is dominated by refined carbohydrate, insulin handling becomes a central issue quickly. When a meal is rich in fat, bile release and slower gastric emptying become more important. When a meal is rich in protein, strong acid secretion and proteolysis matter. Modern mixed foods combine all three, but often in the least coherent proportions. A sugary pastry fried in industrial fat and built on refined flour is a good example. The sugar drives reward and fast absorption. The fat extends mouthfeel and raises energy density. The flour creates an easy starch substrate. Protein is minimal, so the meal delivers little of the amino acid density that would help finish the meal biologically. The eater gets a large energy event with a weak structural signal. That is why such foods often feel filling for a moment but unsatisfying soon after.

The hormonal picture becomes disordered for the same reason. Rapidly absorbed carbohydrate pushes insulin up. Fat slows the digestive timeline. Hyper-palatable texture encourages speed of intake. Weak protein leaves peptide YY and other protein-linked satiety signals underpowered relative to the total energy load. The body can manage this, but management is not the same as alignment. Blood glucose may rise and then fall in a pattern that encourages more eating. Gastric emptying may be slowed just enough to create heaviness without producing the kind of deep satiety that comes from a genuinely nutrient-dense meal. The brain interprets the flavor and texture as highly rewarding while the tissues remain partly unconvinced that enough useful material has arrived. The result is familiar. Cravings, sleepiness, unstable energy, post-meal heaviness, a quick return of hunger, or the strange urge to keep eating even after substantial intake.

This is why mixed modern meals are often harder on appetite than their calorie count suggests. They do not merely add ingredients together. They create a digestive environment in which reward, speed, energy density, and satiety are poorly synchronized. The eater experiences this as a failure of control. The physiology is easier to read. The meal gave the body conflicting instructions, and the body handled them imperfectly because no single digestive program fit the food cleanly. A coherent meal tends to produce a coherent response. A modern industrial meal often produces noise.

Why Some Foods Nourish Cleanly and Others Create Digestive Burden

A food nourishes cleanly when the digestive tract can break it down with relatively little resistance, release useful nutrients in forms that remain available, move those nutrients across the intestinal membrane efficiently, and leave the organs of handling and elimination with a manageable amount of cleanup afterward. A food creates digestive burden when the opposite happens. More mechanical work is required.

More acid, bile, or enzyme output is demanded for less return. Nutrients remain trapped inside structures the body does not dismantle well. Compounds bind minerals before absorption can occur. Fermentable residues reach the colon in amounts that generate distension, gas, osmotic shifts, or irritation. The liver and kidneys are left handling a larger share of what the body could not meaningfully use. The difference is not whether the food sounds wholesome. The difference is whether the organism can turn that food into usable material without paying too much for access.

Animal foods often nourish cleanly because they arrive closer to the chemistry the body is built to process directly. Protein can be denatured by stomach acid, cut by proteases, and reduced to amino acids that match human structural needs closely. Fat can be emulsified by bile and hydrolyzed by lipase into lipid fragments the intestine knows how to absorb. Minerals are often present without the same degree of binding compounds that complicate access in many plant foods. This does not mean every animal food is perfect or every person digests every meal effortlessly. It means the sequence is relatively direct. The body spends digestive effort and usually gets a strong return in amino acids, fats, and bioavailable micronutrients. The food enters, the system recognizes the job, and the yield is high relative to the work required.

Digestive burden tends to rise when food arrives with more structural resistance or more chemical friction. Seeds, grains, legumes, fibrous vegetables, and many processed plant products often carry some combination of cell-wall material, phytate, oxalate, lectins, tannins, resistant starches, or other compounds that slow access, bind nutrients, irritate tissue, or shift more of the meal into microbial fermentation rather than direct absorption. Some of that can be reduced by soaking, sprouting, fermenting, boiling, pressure cooking, peeling, or choosing a less defended plant in the first place. But that need for reduction is already telling you something important. A food that has to be repeatedly modified before it becomes reasonably tolerable is not feeding the organism as cleanly as a food that digestion can process with less negotiation. Preparation can improve yield. It does not erase the fact that the original burden was there.

Processed food creates another kind of digestive burden because it often removes structural resistance in the wrong places while keeping nutritional value weak. Soft starches, refined sugars, industrial fats, emulsifiers, and flavor systems can make a product easy to eat and quick to absorb, but that is not the same as nourishing cleanly. Rapid absorption can flood the system with energy while supplying weak protein, thin micronutrient density, and poor satiety. The digestive burden here is not always a feeling of heaviness or bloating. Sometimes it is regulatory burden. The pancreas has to contain rapid glucose entry. The liver has to process a stream of low-value substrate. Appetite remains active because the meal did not resolve structural need. The food was easy to consume, but hard on the organism in a deeper way. Ease of eating and ease of nourishing are not the same thing.

The colon often reveals the difference clearly. When food nourishes cleanly, less unfinished material reaches the lower gut. Water recovery proceeds, waste forms, and the microbial workload remains in a manageable range. When a meal creates digestive burden, more residue arrives for salvage and fermentation. Gas rises. Distension rises. Transit may speed up or slow down. The person feels bloated, pressured, irritated, or strangely heavy despite having eaten something that was supposed to be healthy. That is not random. It often means the upper digestive tract did not extract enough cleanly, so the lower tract inherited the argument. The colon is then forced to negotiate what the small intestine did not finish.

So the distinction is simple even if the chemistry underneath it is not. Clean nourishment means high yield with relatively low friction. Digestive burden means lower yield with more work, more irritation, more fermentation, more binding, or more downstream disposal cost. The body is not impressed by category reputation. It is measuring what the meal released, what stayed available, what crossed into the body, and what had to be dealt with afterward. That is where the real difference between foods becomes visible.

Chapter 9

Fiber, Antinutrients, and Plant Defense Chemistry

Fiber is usually discussed as if it were a nutrient in the same sense as protein, fat, or a mineral. It is not. Fiber is mostly structural plant material the human digestive system cannot fully break down with its own enzymes. That distinction matters because it changes the entire frame. When the body encounters animal tissue, it can denature proteins, emulsify fats, hydrolyze them into absorbable fragments, and pull useful material across the intestinal lining with relatively direct purpose. When the body encounters fiber, much of what it is meeting is architecture from the plant itself. Cellulose, hemicellulose, lignin, pectin, resistant fractions of starch. These compounds give plants rigidity, water control, and defense. They help the plant stand up, hold shape, protect seeds, and regulate its internal physical structure. But the human small intestine does not possess the enzymatic machinery required to fully dismantle much of that structure and turn it into direct nourishment. Fiber can enter the gut in large quantity and still remain largely inaccessible to the tissues.

This is one reason fiber confuses the nutrition conversation. It has physical effects in the digestive tract, but physical effect is not the same thing as nutritional delivery. Insoluble fiber can increase bulk, change stool form, and mechanically alter transit. Soluble fiber can absorb water, form gels, slow gastric emptying, and alter the rate at which other nutrients contact the absorptive surface. Some fermentable fibers can be used by colonic microbes, which then produce short-chain fatty acids as byproducts. But none of this changes the central fact that fiber itself is not being digested by the human organism in the same direct way that amino acids, fatty acids, glucose, vitamins, and minerals are. It remains, to a large extent, plant scaffolding moving through a digestive tract that can interact with it, but cannot fully access it as food.

That has consequences. A food high in fiber may look substantial on paper while delivering less usable nutrition than its reputation suggests. Bulk can dilute energy density, yes, but it can also dilute access. Fiber can slow contact between digestive enzymes and the nutrients embedded inside the plant matrix. It can trap water, swell in the lumen, and change the mechanical character of the meal without meaningfully increasing the supply of absorbable amino acids, fats, or minerals. In some contexts that may reduce the speed of glucose absorption or alter stool consistency. In other contexts it simply means more material moves through the intestine than the body can actually use. The eater feels full of plant mass. The tissues may still be waiting for real structural input.

The colon is where the human system tries to salvage what it can from this inaccessible material. Microbes ferment some fibers and produce compounds the host can absorb to a limited degree, but this is secondary recovery, not primary nourishment. It is lower-yield, more variable, and more dependent on microbial composition, transit time, and host tolerance than the direct absorption of nutrients in the small intestine. When fiber load rises beyond what the system handles comfortably, the same material often becomes a source of distension, gas, altered motility, and irritation rather than a source of nourishment. That is the deeper point. Fiber is not magic because it changes the contents of the bowel. It is plant structure the body can only partly negotiate. Whether that negotiation helps, hinders, or simply adds bulk depends on dose, form, host condition, and what the fiber displaces from the diet.

Phytic Acid, Lectins, and Other Compounds That Interfere With Digestion

Plant foods are not passive nutrient containers. They are living structures that protect themselves chemically as well as physically, and many of those protective compounds become part of the digestive event once the food is eaten. Phytic acid, lectins, tannins, protease inhibitors, oxalates, saponins, and related compounds do not all behave the same way, but they share an important feature. They complicate access. They either bind nutrients, resist digestion, irritate tissue, interfere with enzymes, or shift more of the meal away from clean absorption and toward friction, salvage, or disposal. This is why a food can test rich in minerals or protein on paper and still nourish poorly in practice. The body is not absorbing the label. It is negotiating with the chemistry that came with the food.

Phytic acid is one of the clearest examples because its main action is binding. Found heavily in seeds, grains, legumes, nuts, and similar plant structures, phytic acid holds phosphorus for the plant and also binds positively charged minerals in the gut. Zinc, iron, calcium, and magnesium can all be trapped in complexes that remain poorly absorbable as the meal moves through the intestine. The nutrient is present, but presence is not delivery. If the mineral stays chemically locked inside the lumen, the body cannot move it across the intestinal membrane in meaningful quantity. This is why a food can appear mineral-rich while behaving like a weak mineral source once digestion becomes real. The food keeps the number. The body loses the access.

Lectins interfere in a different way. They are proteins that can bind to carbohydrates on the surface of cells, including cells lining the intestine. Some are reduced substantially by proper cooking, soaking, fermenting, or pressure cooking, but the need for that reduction already tells you something about the food. In their more active state, lectins can increase digestive friction by interacting with the intestinal surface, altering permeability, irritating local tissue, or interfering with the normal contact between food and absorptive lining. They do not have to create acute poisoning to matter. A smaller repeated interaction at the gut surface is still an interaction. The digestive tract is trying to absorb nutrients across a living membrane. Compounds that bind that membrane or disturb its function change the quality of the event.

Protease inhibitors create yet another problem. These compounds, found especially in many legumes and seeds, interfere with proteases, the enzymes that digest protein. The effect is straightforward. The food may contain protein, but the same food also carries compounds that reduce the body's ability to cut that protein into absorbable amino acids efficiently. Again, label content and biological yield separate. A plant food can be marketed as high protein while simultaneously making access to that protein harder. This is not a philosophical objection. It is a digestive one. The intestine cannot absorb intact complex proteins well. They have to be dismantled first, and anything that impairs that dismantling lowers real value.

Tannins, oxalates, and saponins add more layers of friction. Tannins can bind proteins and reduce digestibility while also interfering with iron absorption. Oxalates can bind calcium and other minerals in the gut and, once absorbed, can shift the burden to the kidney and urinary tract. Saponins can interact with cell membranes and, in some contexts, increase irritation at the intestinal surface. These compounds differ in potency, dose dependence, and host relevance, but together they make the larger point impossible to ignore. Many plant foods do not simply offer nutrients. They offer nutrients mixed with chemistry that can reduce access, raise irritation, or change where the burden lands later in the body.

This is why preparation methods matter so much with plant foods. Soaking, sprouting, fermenting, boiling, and pressure cooking are not culinary decorations. They are attempts to lower chemical defenses, reduce binding activity, improve digestibility, and make the meal less costly to process. Sometimes they help substantially. Sometimes they only reduce the burden rather than remove it. Either way, the need for those steps reveals the underlying biology. A food that repeatedly requires treatment before it becomes reasonably compatible is not behaving like a straightforward nutrient source. It is behaving like defended plant material that humans have learned to work around. That does not make all such foods unusable. It simply means they should be judged by the full digestive sequence, not by reputation or raw composition alone.

Why Plant Foods Often Require Preparation to Reduce Friction

Plant foods often require preparation because the plant is not built to be eaten passively. Its tissues are built to survive long enough to reproduce. Seeds have to protect stored energy and minerals until germination. Leaves have to resist insects, microbes, and grazing. Tubers have to remain intact underground. Legumes have to keep their protein reserve from being consumed before the next generation begins. That means the plant matrix frequently arrives with physical barriers and chemical defenses already in place. Cell walls hold structure. Fibers slow access. Phytic acid binds minerals. Lectins and protease inhibitors interfere with the digestive event. Tannins can bind proteins and reduce digestibility. Oxalates can trap minerals in the gut and, if absorbed, shift burden downstream to the kidney. The body can tolerate some of this, sometimes easily, sometimes poorly, but tolerance is not the same as clean nourishment. Preparation exists because humans have learned, over time, that many plant foods become less obstructive only after they are soaked, peeled, sprouted, fermented, boiled, pressure cooked, ground, or otherwise altered before eating.

The purpose of preparation is therefore not cosmetic. It is mechanical and chemical. Soaking can reduce some soluble compounds and begin softening the matrix. Sprouting changes seed metabolism and can lower portions of the antinutrient burden while altering starch and protein accessibility. Fermentation lets microbes begin part of the dismantling outside the body, lowering some irritants and changing the chemistry of the food before it ever reaches the stomach. Boiling and pressure cooking denature certain heat-sensitive compounds, soften structural barriers, and make starches and proteins more accessible to digestive enzymes. Peeling removes some of the outer defensive tissue where irritating compounds may be concentrated. Grinding increases surface area and breaks open structures the gut would otherwise have to attack more slowly and less completely. Each of these steps is an attempt to shift the digestive event in the body's favor. They are ways of lowering friction before the food enters the human system.

That friction matters because the digestive tract is not a magical solvent that turns every edible thing into nourishment with equal efficiency. The stomach can acidify. The pancreas can release enzymes. Bile can emulsify fat. The small intestine can absorb what becomes available. But none of those powers erase the fact that some foods arrive already closer to usable biology than others. Animal foods generally need breakdown, not neutralization. Many plant foods need both. They need dismantling, and they often need part of their defensive chemistry reduced first. This is why the difference between raw and cooked beans is not a small culinary preference. It is the difference between a food that can be acutely irritating or even toxic in underprepared form and a food that is at least more negotiable after processing. The same principle appears in less dramatic ways across grains, legumes, nuts, tubers, and certain vegetables. Preparation is often the price of entry because the raw food is not offering itself freely.

This is also why preparation should not be mistaken for proof that the food is inherently ideal once processed. Reduction of friction is not the same as elimination of cost. A soaked and cooked grain may be easier to digest than a raw grain, but that does not mean it suddenly delivers the same net yield as a food that began with more accessible protein, more usable fat, and fewer interfering compounds. A pressure-cooked legume may be more tolerable than an undercooked one, but it still may not provide the same protein digestibility, mineral availability, or digestive ease as animal tissue. Preparation can improve compatibility. It cannot fully erase the deeper fact that the food needed substantial intervention before the body could even begin working with it reasonably well. The need for repeated preparation is itself evidence of friction built into the original food.

So when plant foods repeatedly require soaking, sprouting, fermenting, peeling, cooking, or pressure cooking, the right conclusion is not simply that humans are clever cooks. The deeper conclusion is that many plant foods do not meet the human digestive system in their raw state as clean, direct nourishment. They often have to be disarmed first. That does not make them worthless. It makes them conditional. The more a food needs to be modified before it becomes reasonably compatible, the more honestly it should be judged as a food that the body can work around, not a food that naturally feeds the organism with minimal resistance.

Why the Food Label Does Not Tell You What the Intestine Can Actually Extract

A food label describes inventory, not outcome. It tells you what compounds were measured in the product before digestion, but it does not tell you what survives the digestive sequence in usable form, what remains chemically available in the gut lumen, what reaches the absorptive surface of the intestine without being trapped or degraded, and what ultimately crosses into the body. That difference is the beginning of real nutrition. The intestine does not absorb labels. It absorbs molecules that have been released from the food matrix, kept soluble or transportable under gut conditions, and presented to the epithelial membrane in a form transport systems can actually move. A food can test high in protein, iron, calcium, magnesium, or omega-3 fat on paper and still feed the body poorly if those nutrients remain bound, poorly digested, poorly emulsified, poorly transported, or paired with compounds that reduce access before absorption ever begins.

The digestive tract is therefore a filter, not a formality. Protein listed on a package is only potential protein until stomach acid denatures it, proteases cut it, and the small intestine reduces it to amino acids and small peptides that transporters can move across the membrane. Fat listed on a label is only potential fat value until bile acids emulsify it, pancreatic lipase hydrolyzes it, micelles carry the products to the absorptive surface, and intestinal cells reassemble and package those lipids for transport. Minerals listed on a label are especially deceptive because they are vulnerable to gut chemistry. Calcium, iron, zinc, and magnesium do not enter the body simply because they are present in measurable amount. They have to remain available in the intestinal environment. If they bind to phytate, oxalate, fiber-associated compounds, or other interfering molecules, then the number on the label survives while biological delivery falls.

Plant foods make this problem especially visible because many of them package nutrients inside defended structures. A seed may contain minerals and protein, but the same seed may also contain phytic acid that binds those minerals and protease inhibitors that make the protein harder to digest. A leafy plant may test rich in calcium, yet if a large share of that calcium is paired with oxalate, the intestine may extract very little while the rest remains unavailable in the lumen or shifts downstream as a waste-handling problem. A grain product may carry added vitamins and still behave mainly as rapidly available starch with weak satiety and poor structural value. This is why nutrient presence and nutrient yield have to be separated. The label tells you what was detected in the food. The intestine cares about what was liberated, what stayed soluble, and what transport proteins were actually able to move.

Even animal foods, which often perform better in digestibility and bioavailability, still prove the same principle. Their advantage is not that labels suddenly become truth. Their advantage is that the digestive system can usually extract more of what the label is pointing to. Animal protein tends to be more completely digestible. Animal fats tend to be more directly usable. Minerals in animal foods often arrive with less plant-associated binding chemistry. That improves the odds of real absorption, but the governing rule remains the same. The intestine does not read marketing panels. It processes chemistry. The closer a food is to high-yield digestion and absorption, the closer the label comes to reality. The farther the food is from that condition, the more the label becomes a paper promise.

This is why the food label is a weak nutritional authority when used alone. It is useful for rough composition. It is weak for biological accounting. The better question is not what the package says the food contains, but what digestion can actually release from it, what survives interference, what crosses into blood, and what the body is left with after the full event is over.

Part III

Protein as the Primary Structural Input

Chapter 10

Protein as the Structural Language of Biology

Protein is not merely one macronutrient among several. It is the material language of the body's living structure. The body does not build itself out of calories in the abstract. It builds itself out of amino acids arranged into proteins with specific shapes, charges, and functions. Enzymes are proteins. Much of connective tissue is protein. Muscle fibers are protein. Transport molecules in blood are protein. Many receptors at the cell surface are protein. Large parts of the immune response are protein. Even when hormones are not themselves proteins, the enzymes that synthesize, activate, transport, and regulate them usually are. This is why protein sits in a different category from carbohydrate. Carbohydrate may provide fast fuel. Protein provides machinery. It gives the body the raw material required to construct the structures that make life function minute by minute.

Enzymes make this easiest to see. An enzyme is a folded protein that accelerates a chemical reaction the body would otherwise perform too slowly to sustain life. Digestion depends on proteases, lipases, and amylases, each one a protein. Energy production depends on enzyme systems in glycolysis, beta-oxidation, the citric acid cycle, and oxidative phosphorylation, the mitochondrial process that turns nutrient-derived electrons into adenosine triphosphate, or ATP. Detoxification depends on liver enzyme systems that transform compounds into forms the body can excrete. DNA repair, neurotransmitter synthesis, hormone conversion, immune signaling, and mineral handling all depend on protein-based enzymes. If amino acid supply is poor, the body does not simply lose access to a dietary luxury. It begins to strain the very machinery that runs metabolism.

Tissues are built from the same principle. Muscle is the obvious example because it is so visibly protein-rich, but the point runs deeper than muscle size or strength. The intestinal lining turns over rapidly and has to be rebuilt continuously from incoming amino acids. Collagen, the dominant structural protein in connective tissue, holds together skin, tendons, ligaments, fascia, bone matrix, blood vessels, and much of the physical framework that gives the body coherence under tension. Keratin structures hair, nails, and the outer layers of skin. Albumin and other transport proteins move fatty acids, hormones, and minerals through blood. The body is under constant structural maintenance. Proteins are degraded, damaged, oxidized, glycosylated, cleaved, and replaced. A person who thinks about protein only in terms of bodybuilding has already missed the larger biology. The body is always rebuilding itself whether a person is training or not.

Immune function depends on protein in an equally direct way. Antibodies are proteins. Many cytokines, the signaling molecules immune cells use to coordinate defense, are proteins or peptide-derived messengers. Immune receptors that recognize pathogens are protein structures embedded in cellular membranes. Acute-phase proteins produced by the liver rise during infection and inflammation. White blood cells do not defend the body through vague vitality. They defend it through protein-built recognition systems, protein-built signaling cascades, and protein-built effector mechanisms that identify, neutralize, and clear threats. If amino acid availability is chronically poor, immune resilience weakens not as a metaphor but as a material fact. The body has fewer building blocks available for one of its most expensive defense systems.

Hormonal regulation also depends heavily on protein, even though popular discussion often narrows hormones to cholesterol or endocrine glands alone. Many hormones are peptides or proteins, including insulin, glucagon, growth hormone, and a wide range of signaling molecules released by the gut and brain. These do not appear by magic. They are synthesized from amino acids. Even steroid hormones, which are built from cholesterol rather than amino acids, still rely on protein-based receptors, protein transporters, and protein enzymes to be synthesized, activated, and regulated properly. The endocrine system is therefore not separate from protein biology. It is saturated with it. When protein sufficiency falls, hormone signaling does not necessarily collapse in one dramatic moment, but the body begins to operate with less material support for regulatory precision.

Repair is where all of these threads come together. Every day the body is correcting microdamage from ordinary life. Muscle fibers are repaired after movement. Intestinal cells are replaced after frictional and chemical exposure. Skin is rebuilt after abrasion and ultraviolet injury. Liver tissue is renewed after metabolic workload. Blood proteins are resynthesized. Enzymes are replaced. Immune proteins are produced and cleared. None of this can occur without amino acids entering from the diet in adequate quantity and useful balance. The body can recycle some amino acids from old tissue, but recycling is not the same as abundance. When intake is inadequate, the organism begins triage. Less urgent structures wait. Lean tissue may be broken down to support more vital processes. Repair slows. Recovery weakens. The scale may not show the problem immediately, but the physiology already has. Protein is therefore not simply helpful. It is the primary incoming material from which the body keeps itself built, regulated, defended, and repaired.

Essential Amino Acids and Why They Matter

Amino acids are the smaller molecular units from which proteins are built, but they are not all equal from the body's point of view. Some can be produced internally through normal metabolism if enough nitrogen, carbon skeletons, and energy are available. Others cannot. Those are the essential amino acids, the amino acids the human body must obtain from food because it does not have the metabolic machinery to synthesize them in sufficient quantity on its own. That fact changes the whole nutritional question. Protein is not valuable merely because it exists in a food. It is valuable because it carries the specific amino acids the body is unable to make for itself, and it carries them in ratios close enough to human needs that protein synthesis can actually proceed without bottleneck. If even one essential amino acid is short, the body cannot simply improvise the missing part. The machinery slows because the substrate is incomplete.

This matters because the body builds proteins as complete structures, not as approximations. Muscle proteins, digestive enzymes, transport proteins, antibodies, receptors, structural collagen networks, peptide hormones, and countless other protein-based systems require exact amino acid supply. The body can recycle some amino acids from old tissue and can synthesize non-essential amino acids as needed, but it cannot create essential amino acids out of nothing. They have to enter from the diet. That means a food can look high in protein by weight and still underperform biologically if the amino acid pattern is weak, imbalanced, or poorly digested. The issue is not just total grams. The issue is whether the protein arriving in the small intestine actually provides the limiting amino acids in enough quantity to let the body build without interruption. Protein synthesis is constrained by the weakest link. A surplus of several amino acids does not cancel a shortage of one essential one.

Animal foods tend to matter here because they usually provide complete protein, meaning all essential amino acids are present in proportions that match human tissue needs relatively well and in forms digestion can liberate efficiently. Meat, eggs, dairy, and fish do not merely carry protein as a label feature. They carry a more complete instruction set for tissue building. Many plant foods do contain amino acids, sometimes in respectable total amounts, but their profiles are often less aligned with human structural demand, and the proteins are more likely to be packaged with fiber, antinutrients, or protease inhibitors that reduce real yield. The result is that total intake and usable intake begin to separate. The food number stays high. The body still has to work harder to get less.

Leucine is a useful example because it is not only essential, it also functions as a nutrient signal. When enough leucine reaches tissues, particularly muscle, it helps activate pathways involved in protein synthesis. In practical terms, that means certain foods do not just provide raw material. They also help tell the body that the raw material is sufficient for building to proceed. This is one reason protein quality matters so much in the real world. A meal weak in essential amino acids may deliver energy and some nitrogen while failing to create a strong repair signal. A meal rich in complete protein can do both at once. The body receives substrate and permission.

Essential amino acids therefore matter because they draw a hard line between what the body can tolerate and what the body can actually build from. They are not optional details inside the protein story. They are the reason protein has to be judged by quality, digestibility, and usable composition rather than by raw quantity alone. The body is constantly rebuilding itself. It cannot do that honestly with missing pieces.

Why the Body Has No Large Reserve Pool of Amino Acids

The body stores energy easily. It stores glycogen in liver and muscle. It stores triglycerides in adipose tissue. It stores minerals to varying degrees in bone and other tissues. Protein is different. The body does not maintain a large free-floating warehouse of amino acids waiting to be drawn down at leisure because amino acids are not mainly an energy reserve. They are active structural material. Once amino acids enter circulation, the body tends to use them, incorporate them into proteins, convert them, or clear their nitrogen rather than hold them in a large idle pool. Free amino acids are maintained in a relatively small circulating and intracellular supply, enough to support ongoing turnover and immediate synthesis, but not enough to function as a deep reserve comparable to body fat. That is the first point. Protein is not stockpiled in the body as spare parts lying around untouched. It is built into living tissue.

That design makes sense once protein is understood for what it is. Amino acids are the raw material for enzymes, muscle fibers, transport proteins, peptide hormones, immune molecules, collagen, gut lining turnover, and countless repair processes. These molecules are useful when assembled into functioning structures, not when left loose in bulk. A large reserve pool of free amino acids would also create chemical handling problems. Amino acids contain nitrogen, and nitrogen handling is tightly regulated because excess free nitrogen becomes ammonia, which is toxic, especially to the nervous system. The liver can convert ammonia into urea for excretion, but that is a disposal pathway, not a storage strategy. The body therefore avoids treating amino acids like long-term bulk inventory. When intake exceeds immediate synthetic need, the surplus is often oxidized for energy, converted into other compounds, or deaminated and cleared rather than banked indefinitely as a free amino acid stash.

This is why muscle sometimes gets misunderstood as a protein storage site. Muscle is not a passive pantry built for convenient withdrawal. It is functional tissue. It stores protein only in the sense that it is made of protein, and under stress, starvation, illness, or chronically inadequate intake, the body can break it down to recover amino acids for more urgent needs. That is an emergency borrowing system, not a preferred design. When dietary protein is insufficient, the body begins pulling from its own structure to maintain immune function, enzyme turnover, glucose production when needed, and other vital processes. The organism is not drawing from a generous reserve pool. It is cannibalizing working tissue. That is why low protein intake can gradually show up as weakness, poor recovery, thinning lean mass, reduced resilience, and slower repair even when calories remain adequate. Energy can be stored cheaply. Structure cannot.

The absence of a large amino acid reserve also explains why regular protein intake matters so much more than people assume. The body is in constant turnover. Intestinal cells are replaced rapidly. Enzymes degrade and are rebuilt. Immune proteins are synthesized and cleared. Muscle proteins are continuously remodeled. Connective tissue is maintained. Skin renews. None of this pauses because intake was low for a while. The organism keeps spending amino acids whether the diet replenishes them or not. Since there is no deep free reserve to draw from, protein sufficiency depends on repeated supply. The body can recycle some amino acids from old proteins, and that recycling is important, but recycling is not enough to cover everything indefinitely. New input still has to arrive.

This is one of the main reasons protein sits in a different category from carbohydrate. The body can make glucose when it needs to. It cannot make essential amino acids. It can store large amounts of fat. It cannot store large amounts of free amino acids without turning living tissue into the storage medium itself. So when protein is underfed, the cost is structural. The body does not simply feel a little low on a dietary target. It starts losing the materials it uses to keep itself built.

Nitrogen Balance and the Cost of Inadequate Protein Intake

Nitrogen balance is one of the clearest ways to understand why protein is not optional background nutrition. Amino acids are distinguished from fat and carbohydrate by the presence of nitrogen. That nitrogen is what allows them to be built into proteins, enzymes, transport molecules, immune factors, and other living structures the body cannot make from glucose or fatty acids alone. Nitrogen balance is the relationship between how much nitrogen enters the body through dietary protein and how much leaves the body through urine, stool, sweat, skin loss, and other routes. When intake is sufficient to cover ongoing turnover, repair, immune demand, enzyme replacement, and tissue maintenance, the body can remain in nitrogen equilibrium. When intake falls below need, the body enters negative nitrogen balance. That does not mean a theoretical deficiency on paper. It means the organism is losing more protein-derived material than it is replacing. Since the body has no large reserve pool of free amino acids, it solves that gap by drawing from itself.

That cost is structural before it is visible. Muscle is often the easiest place to notice it, but muscle is only one tissue paying the bill. The body may begin breaking down contractile proteins to recover amino acids for more urgent uses such as immune function, glucose production when needed, acute repair, and maintenance of critical organs. But the drain does not stop there. Intestinal cells turn over rapidly and require constant protein supply. Digestive enzymes have to be resynthesized. Plasma proteins that transport hormones, fats, and minerals have to be maintained. Collagen and other connective tissue proteins need ongoing renewal. The immune system builds antibodies, receptors, cytokines, and acute-phase proteins from amino acid substrate. A chronically low-protein intake therefore does not merely make someone a little less anabolic. It forces the body into triage. Less essential tissues and functions begin absorbing the damage so more essential ones can continue.

The body can hide this for a while, which is one reason inadequate protein intake is so often underestimated. Weight may remain stable if total calories are sufficient. A person may even lose fat for a period and interpret the result as nutritional success. But negative nitrogen balance can still be running underneath that visual outcome. Recovery becomes weaker. Lean mass is harder to maintain. Strength plateaus or falls. Hair and skin quality may worsen. Satiety becomes less reliable. Immune resilience weakens. Wound healing slows. The person often experiences this not as a dramatic deficiency syndrome but as a general flattening of structural competence. The body is still operating, but it is doing so while economizing on the very material it uses to keep itself intact.

The liver reveals another part of the story. Amino acids that are not used immediately for synthesis can be deaminated, meaning their nitrogen group is removed. That nitrogen is converted into urea through the urea cycle and excreted by the kidneys. When protein intake is adequate, this system helps regulate amino acid turnover cleanly. When intake is inadequate, however, the issue is not excess nitrogen disposal but insufficient nitrogen availability for building. The body cannot create essential amino acids out of stored fat or carbohydrate. It cannot pay back a chronic protein debt with better glucose control or lower calorie intake. It either receives enough nitrogen-containing substrate to maintain protein synthesis, or it starts dismantling existing proteins to keep critical pathways alive.

This is why nitrogen balance matters more than most people realize. It exposes the difference between being fueled and being maintained. A person can have enough calories to keep body weight from collapsing while still lacking enough protein to preserve structure over time. Energy sufficiency does not guarantee protein sufficiency. The body may remain alive, but it does so by consuming pieces of itself. That is the real cost of inadequate protein intake. It is not only hunger, weakness, or a missed fitness target. It is a quiet withdrawal from the tissues, enzymes, and repair systems that keep the organism well built.

Chapter 11

Protein Digestion and Amino Acid Extraction

Protein digestion does not begin in the stomach. It begins when the body recognizes that food, especially substantial food, is about to arrive. Sight, smell, anticipation, chewing, and taste all feed into what physiology calls the cephalic phase, the early neural stage of digestion in which the brain begins preparing the digestive tract before the meal has fully entered it. This preparation is not decorative. It changes the quality of the entire digestive event. Saliva rises. The stomach begins increasing acid secretion. Gastrin signaling starts to build. The pancreas is primed. Motility shifts. The gut is told that incoming material is likely to require real dismantling rather than simple passage. This matters most with protein because protein is structurally demanding. It arrives as folded chains that cannot be absorbed intact and cannot be used until the body has unfolded them, cut them down, and moved the resulting amino acids or short peptides across the intestinal lining. The cephalic phase is therefore the body's first investment in making that possible.

The mouth contributes more than mechanical reduction. Chewing breaks food into smaller particles, increasing exposed surface area so acid and enzymes can work more efficiently later. That seems obvious, but it is easy to underestimate how important it is when eating is rushed. Large poorly chewed pieces of meat or other dense protein foods reach the stomach as harder chemical targets. They require more time, more acid exposure, and more mechanical churning before the proteins are sufficiently denatured. Saliva does not digest protein in the way gastric and pancreatic enzymes do, but it still matters because it lubricates the bolus, coordinates swallowing, and helps synchronize the rest of the tract through neural signaling. In effect, the mouth tells the stomach what kind of workload is approaching. Fast, distracted eating weakens that conversation. The meal still enters. The system is simply less prepared when it does.

Once the cephalic phase is active, the stomach is already shifting into a high-acid, protein-oriented state before the full digestive burden arrives. Parietal cells begin secreting hydrochloric acid. Chief cells prepare pepsinogen, the inactive precursor that becomes pepsin in an acidic environment. Gastrin supports both secretion and gastric motility, helping turn the stomach into a controlled protein-processing chamber rather than a holding bag. This is important because protein digestion depends on sequence. First the structure has to be exposed. Then enzymes can cut. Then the resulting fragments can be delivered in manageable amounts to the small intestine, where pancreatic proteases and brush-border enzymes continue the dismantling. If the early phase is weak, the downstream work becomes less efficient. The stomach may underacidify. Protein may sit heavier. Larger fragments may move forward before they have been properly prepared. The problem then appears later as poor digestion, bloating, fullness, or weak amino acid extraction, but part of the failure began upstream in preparation.

This is why digestive readiness matters more than most people realize. Protein is not a passive nutrient that drifts into the body because it was eaten. It has to be received by a system that was given time to organize itself around the task. The cephalic phase is the body's way of doing that. It is the first move in a chain that ends with amino acids entering the bloodstream and becoming enzymes, muscle proteins, immune molecules, transport proteins, and repair material. When that first move is strong, the rest of the sequence has a better chance of running cleanly. When it is weak, the entire protein digestion process begins with less coordination and more friction.

Stomach Acid and Protein Denaturation

Stomach acid is not a harsh accessory to digestion. It is one of the first major tools the body uses to convert food protein into something biologically usable. Protein arrives in food as a folded structure. Muscle tissue, connective tissue, enzymes inside the food itself, albumins, globulins, all of them are built from amino acid chains bent and packed into specific three-dimensional forms. Those forms are stable enough to serve life inside the animal or plant they came from, but they are not directly absorbable by the human intestine. Before the body can extract amino acids from them, those structures have to be opened. That is what stomach acid begins to do. Hydrochloric acid lowers gastric pH to a highly acidic range, often around 1.5 to 3, and that acidity disrupts the bonds that hold protein in its folded shape. The protein does not vanish. It unfolds. This is denaturation. The chain remains there, but the protective architecture around it begins to collapse.

That unfolding matters because digestive enzymes do not cut proteins efficiently when the peptide backbone is still buried inside tight folded structure. Denaturation exposes more of the chain to enzymatic attack. It takes a biologically functional protein and turns it into a vulnerable substrate. Once the protein is opened, pepsin can begin cleaving it into smaller fragments. Pepsin itself depends on the same acidic environment because it is secreted as pepsinogen, an inactive precursor that only becomes active under low pH conditions. This means stomach acid is doing two jobs at once. It is changing the food, and it is activating the tool that will cut the changed food. Without sufficient acid, protein stays more structurally intact and pepsin activity falls. The entire downstream sequence becomes weaker because the small intestine receives material that was not properly prepared upstream.

This is one reason protein-rich meals create a different gastric event than meals dominated by refined carbohydrate. The stomach is not just filling with food. It is entering a high-acid, protein-processing state. Gastrin rises, acid output rises, and the meal is churned against that acid until more of its structure is chemically exposed. Connective tissue softens. Muscle proteins lose their tight form. Pepsin begins the first stage of proteolysis, the cutting of proteins into smaller peptide fragments. The stomach is therefore not simply a holding chamber. It is the first major site where dietary protein is turned from tissue into digestible substrate.

Acid also contributes to microbial control. Food does not arrive sterile, and animal foods in particular historically carried meaningful microbial exposure risk. A highly acidic stomach reduces that burden before food moves deeper into the tract. This is not separate from protein digestion. It is part of the same gastric logic. A system built to handle dense protein foods benefits from strong acid because strong acid both opens protein structure and reduces the survival of unwanted organisms traveling with the meal. The same chemistry that prepares nourishment also protects the host.

When stomach acid is inadequate, the cost is not abstract. Protein digestion becomes less efficient. Heavy meals may sit longer. Larger fragments may pass forward before proper denaturation and early cleavage have occurred. The person may feel fullness, pressure, reflux-like discomfort, or the vague sense that dense protein foods do not sit well, when the deeper problem is that the stomach never fully entered the acid state needed to process them cleanly. The small intestine and pancreas can continue the work later, but they are being handed a meal that was insufficiently prepared. Protein digestion begins there, but it begins badly.

This is why stomach acid matters so much in any serious discussion of protein nutrition. A food can contain abundant protein, and the label can look impressive, but until the stomach has denatured that protein and activated the first proteolytic step, the amino acids are still locked inside folded biological structure. The stomach does not merely acidify food because acid is present in the body. It acidifies food because structure has to be broken before nourishment can begin.

Pancreatic Proteases and Brush Border Digestion

Stomach acid begins protein digestion, but it does not finish it. By the time chyme leaves the stomach, most dietary protein has only been denatured and cut into smaller peptide fragments. The heavy structural work has started, but the amino acids are still locked inside chains too large to cross the intestinal membrane. The next major stage takes place in the small intestine, and it depends on the pancreas. As acidic chyme enters the duodenum, bicarbonate from the pancreas neutralizes the gastric acid enough to protect the intestinal lining and create the pH range in which pancreatic enzymes can function properly. At the same time, the pancreas releases proteases, protein-digesting enzymes, in inactive forms so they do not digest pancreatic tissue before they reach the gut lumen. Once in the intestine, those enzymes are activated and begin dismantling the peptide fragments that survived the stomach.

Trypsin is one of the central enzymes in this stage. It is released as trypsinogen and activated in the small intestine by enteropeptidase, an enzyme located at the intestinal surface. Once active, trypsin does not work alone. It activates other pancreatic proteases as well, including chymotrypsin, elastase, and carboxypeptidases. Each of these enzymes cuts peptide chains at different points. Some target internal bonds next to particular amino acids. Others trim amino acids from the ends of peptides. The result is controlled reduction. Large peptide fragments become smaller peptides, then smaller still. This matters because digestion is not random destruction. It is staged disassembly. The pancreas is taking the denatured, partially hydrolyzed protein material delivered by the stomach and reducing it into forms the intestinal surface can finish.

The brush border is where that finishing work happens. The brush border is the dense microscopic surface of the small intestine formed by microvilli, tiny projections that massively expand absorptive area and carry membrane-bound enzymes. These are not background details. They are the final contact zone between dietary protein and the body. Peptidases at the brush border trim the remaining small peptides into free amino acids, dipeptides, and tripeptides, two- and three-amino-acid fragments small enough to be transported into intestinal cells. In some cases, those tiny peptides are absorbed directly and broken down further inside the enterocyte, the absorptive cell lining the intestine. In other words, digestion is completed right at the threshold of entry. The brush border does not merely absorb what is already ready. It creates readiness at the membrane itself.

This is where protein digestion becomes real in biological terms. A food may have contained large amounts of protein, and the stomach may have begun the dismantling, but until pancreatic proteases and brush border enzymes have done their work, the amino acid value remains partly trapped inside peptide structure. The intestine cannot absorb intact meat proteins or intact plant proteins as such. It needs small units. That is why impaired pancreatic output, poor small intestinal health, or damage to the brush border can reduce the real value of protein intake even when the diet looks adequate on paper. The person may be eating enough protein by weight and still extracting too little because the cutting process was incomplete. Label content and absorbed amino acid yield separate at this stage very easily.

This is also one reason animal protein often performs so well biologically. Once its structure has been opened by acid and processed through the pancreatic and brush border sequence, the resulting amino acids tend to arrive in complete, usable patterns that match human structural needs closely. The digestive system still has to do the work, but the payoff is high. The body receives substrate it can actually build with. Pancreatic proteases and brush border digestion are the decisive middle steps in that transfer. They turn food protein into absorbable amino acid material, and without them the body is left with fragments instead of building blocks.

Amino Acid Absorption and Transport

Once protein has been denatured in the stomach, cut by pancreatic proteases in the small intestine, and trimmed at the brush border into free amino acids, dipeptides, and tripeptides, the next question is no longer how to digest it. The question becomes how to get it into the body. This is where absorption begins, and absorption is not passive leakage. The intestinal lining is selective. It is built from epithelial cells that act as controlled gatekeepers between the gut lumen and the bloodstream. Amino acids do not simply drift across because they are small enough. They are moved through specific transport systems embedded in the membrane of enterocytes, the absorptive cells lining the small intestine. Some transporters move single amino acids. Others handle small peptides. Many depend on sodium gradients or hydrogen ion gradients to pull these molecules inward. This means amino acid absorption is not merely a matter of presence. It is an energy-dependent transfer event carried out by living tissue that has to recognize, bind, and move the products of digestion across a barrier.

The brush border does part of the last digestive work at the same time. Some amino acids are absorbed directly as free amino acids, but a significant share of protein digestion products enters the enterocyte as dipeptides and tripeptides. These short chains are carried through dedicated peptide transporters and then broken down further inside the cell by intracellular peptidases. That detail matters because it shows how tightly digestion and absorption are linked. The intestine is not waiting for the lumen to produce perfect purity before it acts. It finishes the job at the point of transfer. The result is that what began as muscle tissue, collagen, albumin, or other dietary protein is progressively reduced into amino acid units the body can actually claim as its own. The food is becoming internal, but only through a membrane system that demands precision at every step.

Once amino acids cross the intestinal cell, they do not go directly to muscle or other peripheral tissues first. Most of them leave the intestine through the portal circulation and are delivered straight to the liver. This is one of the most important control points in protein metabolism. The liver receives the first wave of absorbed amino acids and decides what portion will be retained, transformed, stored transiently in metabolic pathways, converted into other compounds, or released into the broader circulation. It may use some amino acids for its own protein synthesis and enzyme production. It may convert nitrogen into urea when amino acid breakdown is occurring. It may direct carbon skeletons toward gluconeogenesis, the endogenous production of glucose from non-carbohydrate substrates, if metabolic conditions require it. What remains is then passed outward into the bloodstream where other tissues can draw from the circulating amino acid pool. This means amino acid transport is not just about crossing the intestine. It is about entering a managed distribution system.

That circulating amino acid pool is relatively small, but it is metabolically vital. Muscle draws from it for repair and turnover. The immune system draws from it for antibodies, cytokines, and rapidly expanding cell populations during challenge. The gut itself draws from it because intestinal tissue renews quickly and depends heavily on constant substrate supply. The skin, liver, endocrine system, connective tissue, and nervous system all depend on amino acid traffic moving through blood in usable form. This is why absorption efficiency matters so much. If digestion is incomplete, if transport at the intestinal surface is impaired, or if the protein source is poorly digestible and yields fewer absorbable fragments, then the problem is not simply that the meal was imperfect. The problem is that the body receives less building material into the shared pool that sustains ongoing repair and regulation. The food entered the mouth. The tissues still did not receive the full value.

This is also why protein quality and digestive health cannot be separated. A food may carry high protein on paper, but if its amino acids are poorly liberated, poorly transported, or delivered in an imbalanced pattern, the bloodstream does not see that labeled value. The intestine only transfers what digestion has made available and what the membrane system can handle. The body then only builds from what circulation actually receives. Amino acid absorption and transport are therefore the decisive conversion point where protein stops being food and becomes biological material. Everything before this stage is preparation. Everything after it is construction.

Liver Handling of Incoming Amino Acids

Once amino acids cross the intestinal lining, they do not enter the body as a free gift delivered equally to every tissue. They go first to the liver through the portal circulation, and that first pass matters because the liver is the body's primary sorting organ. It sits between absorption and distribution, deciding what portion of the incoming amino acid load will be used locally, what will be transformed, what will be released into general circulation, and what will be broken down because it exceeds immediate structural demand. This means the liver is not a passive checkpoint. It is the first major authority the body uses to interpret what protein intake actually means metabolically. A meal rich in amino acids has arrived. The question is no longer whether digestion succeeded. The question is how that amino acid influx will be allocated.

Part of that allocation is straightforward tissue maintenance. The liver is a protein-intensive organ. It is constantly synthesizing enzymes, transport proteins, clotting factors, albumin, acute-phase proteins involved in inflammation and immune defense, and a wide range of regulatory molecules that keep blood chemistry stable. Albumin alone, the major transport protein in blood plasma, is a good example of why this matters. It binds and carries fatty acids, hormones, bilirubin, drugs, and other compounds through circulation. That protein has to be made somewhere, and the liver makes it from incoming amino acids. The same is true for many enzymes involved in detoxification, glucose handling, ammonia disposal, and lipid metabolism. So the first thing the liver does with absorbed amino acids is not to count them as calories. It asks what it needs to keep its own machinery running.

The liver also acts as a conversion site. Some amino acids can be used directly for protein synthesis. Others can be transaminated, meaning their amino group is transferred to another carbon skeleton so the body can generate different non-essential amino acids according to need. This is one reason amino acid metabolism is more dynamic than people realize. The liver is not just a warehouse releasing amino acids unchanged. It is reshaping part of the amino acid traffic so the rest of the organism can receive the right mix of substrates. This conversion work depends on enzymes, vitamin cofactors, and intact hepatic function. When the liver handles amino acids well, the body gets not only what the meal directly provided but also a regulated downstream supply adapted to immediate physiological priorities.

Nitrogen handling is another central task. Amino acids are valuable because they contain nitrogen, but that same nitrogen becomes a problem when amino acids are broken down beyond what is needed for synthesis. The carbon skeleton may be used for energy, glucose production, or other metabolic pathways, but the nitrogen group cannot simply accumulate. Free ammonia is toxic, especially to the nervous system. The liver solves this through the urea cycle, a controlled biochemical pathway that converts ammonia into urea, a safer compound that can travel in the blood to the kidneys for excretion. This means the liver is constantly deciding whether incoming amino acids are being routed toward building or toward breakdown, and if breakdown occurs, it must manage the nitrogen burden carefully. Protein is therefore never just structure or just energy. The liver determines which side of that balance dominates after the meal.

This is also where gluconeogenesis enters the picture. When carbohydrate intake is low or metabolic demand shifts, the liver can take certain amino acid carbon skeletons and convert them into glucose. That does not mean protein exists mainly to become sugar. It means the liver preserves metabolic flexibility by using amino acids when necessary to maintain blood glucose for tissues that require it. This is an adaptive feature, but it also reinforces the hierarchy of protein use. The body would rather use amino acids for repair, enzymes, immune proteins, and tissue maintenance first. Glucose production from amino acids is a real pathway, but it is not the reason protein is nutritionally important. It is part of the liver's ability to keep the organism stable under changing conditions.

So the liver's handling of incoming amino acids reveals something essential about protein biology. Absorption is not the end of the story. The liver receives the first shipment, claims what it needs, reshapes part of the supply, disposes of excess nitrogen, and only then releases amino acids into wider circulation for muscle, immune tissue, connective tissue, endocrine signaling, and ongoing repair elsewhere. Protein becomes biologically useful only because this sorting process is disciplined. Without the liver, amino acid traffic would be chemically dangerous and metabolically chaotic. With it, dietary protein is turned into ordered structural supply.

What Happens When Protein Digestion Fails

When protein digestion fails, the problem is not abstract. The body loses access to one of its main structural inputs while the person may still believe he is eating enough. A plate can contain plenty of protein on paper and still deliver too little in practice if the digestive sequence breaks early. Stomach acid may be too weak to denature protein properly. Pepsin may not activate with enough force. Pancreatic proteases may not arrive in sufficient quantity. Brush-border digestion at the intestinal surface may be impaired. Transit may be poorly timed. The intestinal lining may be inflamed, irritated, or simply less capable of clean absorption. In each case the label stays the same. The body gets less. That gap matters because protein is not mainly a comfort nutrient or a bonus macronutrient. It is the raw material for enzymes, transport proteins, immune molecules, connective tissue, muscle maintenance, gut lining turnover, and repair across the organism.

The first consequence is often local. A person may feel heaviness after protein-rich meals, prolonged fullness, bloating, upper abdominal pressure, burping, or the sense that meat sits in the stomach rather than being processed. Those symptoms are not always caused by protein itself. Often they reflect poor preparation of the meal in the stomach or weak dismantling downstream. If hydrochloric acid is insufficient, proteins remain less denatured and pepsin activity falls. Larger protein fragments then move into the small intestine before they have been properly prepared. The pancreas and brush border are forced to finish a job that started badly. When they cannot fully compensate, digestion becomes inefficient and the meal can feel like work instead of nourishment.

The second consequence is nutritional, and it is more serious because it can remain less visible for longer. If amino acids are not being extracted efficiently, the body has less substrate available for ongoing protein synthesis even when total intake looks respectable. Recovery weakens. Lean mass becomes harder to maintain. The gut lining, which turns over rapidly and depends heavily on amino acid supply, may repair less efficiently. Immune resilience can soften because antibodies, cytokines, receptors, and acute-phase proteins all depend on protein substrate. Wound healing slows. Hair, nails, skin, and connective tissues may begin showing subtle loss of structural quality. A person may be fully capable of consuming enough calories while quietly underdelivering the amino acids required to keep the organism built.

The body then begins compensating, and compensation has a cost. Since there is no large reserve pool of free amino acids, the organism may begin drawing more heavily from its own tissues to cover essential needs. Muscle becomes one source, but not the only one. This is the deeper danger of failed protein digestion. The person may not look starved. He may even be carrying excess body fat. But metabolically he is still running a structural deficit. The body can burn carbohydrate and fat for fuel. It cannot manufacture essential amino acids when intake and extraction are inadequate. So it starts economizing, borrowing, and triaging. Less urgent repair waits. More urgent survival functions are protected. The outside story may still sound like "I eat plenty." The inside story has already changed.

Another consequence is that more unfinished protein can move further down the gut than it should. The small intestine is built to absorb amino acids and very small peptides, not large quantities of incompletely digested protein material. When too much escapes earlier processing, microbial interactions and digestive discomfort often rise. That can mean more fermentation-like symptoms, more foul-smelling gas, more intestinal irritation, or a greater sense that meals are creating residue rather than clean nourishment. The colon then inherits part of a workload that should have been finished upstream. What reaches the lower gut says something important about what earlier stages failed to extract.

This is why protein digestion has to be protected, not assumed. Adequate stomach acid, coordinated pancreatic enzyme release, intact bile flow where fat-protein meals are involved, healthy brush-border function, and a reasonably intact intestinal lining are not optional details. They are part of whether protein-rich food becomes amino acid supply or simply passes through as partially used material. When protein digestion fails, the body does not merely miss out on a dietary preference. It loses access to the very substrate it uses to keep itself repaired, regulated, defended, and structurally intact.

Chapter 12

Protein Quality, Bioavailability, and Muscle Maintenance

A protein source is complete when it delivers all of the essential amino acids in amounts and proportions that allow the body to build without running into a limiting shortage. It is incomplete when one or more of those essential amino acids are too low to support efficient protein synthesis on their own. That difference sounds technical, but it reaches directly into tissue maintenance. The body does not assemble muscle, enzymes, immune proteins, transport molecules, and connective tissue from a vague cloud of "protein." It assembles them from specific amino acids, and essential amino acids have to arrive from food because the body cannot manufacture them in sufficient quantity internally. If one of them is missing or too low, the whole building process slows. This is why total grams of protein can mislead. A food may carry a respectable protein number and still function as a weaker structural input because the amino acid pattern is incomplete.

Animal foods matter here because they tend to arrive already aligned with human protein needs. Meat, eggs, fish, and dairy generally contain the full essential amino acid spectrum in ratios that more closely match what human tissues repeatedly require. Once digestion has done its work, the resulting amino acid pool gives the body a cleaner instruction set for synthesis. Muscle repair, enzyme turnover, immune signaling, and connective tissue maintenance can proceed without the same degree of bottleneck. That is what complete protein really means in biological terms. It does not mean a food is morally superior or magically anabolic. It means the food delivers the full amino acid pattern needed to support protein synthesis with less compromise and less need for compensatory food combining.

Incomplete protein creates a different situation. Many plant foods contain protein, sometimes in substantial amounts by weight, but the amino acid pattern is often skewed. One food may be relatively low in lysine. Another may be weaker in methionine. Another may contain protein that is technically present but less accessible because it is bound inside fibrous structure or paired with protease inhibitors and other interfering compounds. The body can still use what is available, but the synthesis ceiling is lower when the amino acid pattern is unbalanced. A surplus of some amino acids does not erase the shortage of another. Protein synthesis is constrained by the limiting amino acid, the essential amino acid present in the shortest supply relative to the body's need. Once that limiting factor is reached, more of the non-limiting amino acids do not solve the problem. The meal may still contribute something. It simply does not perform like a complete structural input on its own.

This is why the conversation has to move beyond protein quantity and into protein quality. Two meals can contain the same nominal grams of protein and still differ sharply in what the body can build from them. One may provide a complete, highly digestible amino acid pattern that supports muscle maintenance and broader protein turnover cleanly. The other may require larger volume, more total calories, more digestive work, or strategic combining with other foods before it approaches the same functional result. That does not mean incomplete proteins are useless. It means they should be judged honestly. The body does not care whether the label says "high protein." It cares whether the amino acid profile, digestibility, and net absorption are sufficient to support actual synthesis once the meal is over.

Why Animal Protein Aligns More Closely With Human Requirements

Animal protein aligns more closely with human requirements because the body is trying to build human tissue, not merely process nitrogen. That distinction is the center of the issue. A protein source is valuable to the extent that digestion can liberate its amino acids and those amino acids arrive in proportions that fit the recurring demands of human structure. Muscle repair, enzyme turnover, connective tissue maintenance, immune protein synthesis, gut lining renewal, transport proteins, peptide hormones, all of these processes require a full essential amino acid pattern delivered in usable balance. Animal foods tend to provide that balance more directly because animal tissue is already built from protein structures much closer to the body's own needs. Once digestion breaks meat, eggs, fish, or dairy down into amino acids, the resulting pool more often resembles what the human organism is repeatedly trying to make. That does not eliminate digestion. It means the payoff from digestion is usually more coherent.

This alignment matters because protein quality is not just about the presence of amino acids. It is about the relative proportion of essential amino acids, digestibility, and how much of the absorbed material can actually be turned into human protein without one limiting amino acid slowing the entire process. Animal proteins generally contain all essential amino acids in amounts that support synthesis more efficiently than most plant proteins do on their own. Many plant proteins are lower in one or more essential amino acids relative to human demand, and that shortage becomes the bottleneck. The body cannot build a complete protein structure from enthusiasm and extra carbohydrate. It has to have the full amino acid set. If lysine, methionine, leucine, or another essential amino acid is underdelivered relative to need, the rest of the amino acid pool cannot fully compensate. The synthesis signal weakens because the substrate is incomplete.

Digestibility sharpens the same point. Animal proteins are usually easier for the human digestive system to denature, cleave, and absorb with high efficiency. Stomach acid unfolds them. Pepsin begins cutting them. Pancreatic proteases and brush-border enzymes finish the reduction into amino acids and small peptides. The intestine then transports those products across the membrane into circulation. Many plant proteins, by contrast, arrive packaged inside fibrous structures or alongside protease inhibitors, lectins, tannins, and other compounds that can reduce digestibility or interfere with extraction. So the issue is not only that the amino acid profile may be weaker. The issue is that the body often has to work through more friction to obtain a less complete result. The food can still be eaten. The yield is often lower.

Leucine is one useful example because it shows that protein quality is both structural and regulatory. Leucine is an essential amino acid that helps activate muscle protein synthesis and signals that sufficient building material is available. Animal proteins tend to deliver leucine in amounts that help support this signaling more effectively per serving than many plant proteins do. That means a meal built around animal protein often does two things at once. It supplies the raw material and strengthens the instruction to build. A weaker protein source may provide some amino acids without creating the same threshold effect. This is one reason equal grams of protein do not always create equal biological outcomes.

The body also pays a cost when it has to obtain protein through larger food volume and lower protein density. If a person has to eat far more carbohydrate, far more fiber, or far more total food just to approximate the amino acid delivery of a smaller amount of animal protein, the protein question is no longer isolated. Digestive burden rises. Appetite regulation changes. Glucose handling changes. Mineral absorption may become more complicated. The larger meal may still fail to match the digestibility and essential amino acid sufficiency of the smaller animal-food meal. That is why alignment matters. It is not an abstract ranking system. It changes what the body actually receives, how much work the digestive tract has to do, and what tissue maintenance looks like over time.

So when animal protein is said to align more closely with human requirements, the claim is not mystical or ideological. It is anatomical, digestive, and biochemical. The human body needs a full essential amino acid pattern, delivered in forms digestion can access efficiently, in quantities sufficient to support continuous repair and renewal. Animal protein tends to meet that demand more directly, with less dilution, less interference, and less need for compensation. That is what alignment means in real physiology.

Leucine Threshold and Muscle Protein Synthesis

Muscle protein synthesis does not rise simply because some protein was eaten. It rises when a meal delivers enough digestible essential amino acids, and especially enough leucine, to convince the body that real building material has arrived in sufficient concentration to justify turning repair machinery on. Leucine is one of the branched-chain amino acids, but its importance is not just that it becomes part of muscle tissue. It also acts as a nutrient signal. When leucine appears in the bloodstream in adequate quantity after digestion, it helps activate mTOR, short for mechanistic target of rapamycin, a central cellular pathway that tells muscle cells conditions are favorable for protein synthesis. That pathway does not respond strongly to intention, appetite, or protein branding. It responds to substrate. If the meal fails to deliver enough leucine and enough of the other essential amino acids alongside it, the building signal stays weak even if the eater believes he consumed a respectable amount of protein.

This is why threshold matters. Muscle protein synthesis behaves less like a dimmer switch that rises smoothly with every extra gram and more like a system that needs a sufficient trigger before it responds meaningfully. A meal can contain some protein and still underperform because the amino acid rise in blood never reaches the point where muscle tissue interprets the event as a genuine repair opportunity. That is especially important with lower-quality proteins or with meals diluted by carbohydrate and fiber that spread protein thinly across a large food volume. The person may feel full, may have eaten a high-calorie meal, and may even think the meal was protein rich because the label says so, yet the leucine signal may remain too small to create a strong anabolic response. The food entered the stomach. The signal to build never fully arrived.

Animal proteins tend to perform well here because they combine high digestibility with a stronger leucine density and a full essential amino acid pattern. Once stomach acid denatures them, pancreatic proteases and brush-border enzymes reduce them, and the intestine absorbs the resulting amino acids, the bloodstream sees a sharper and more useful amino acid rise. Muscle tissue then receives not just building material, but a coherent signal that enough building material is present to justify synthesis. Many plant proteins struggle at this step for two reasons at once. Their amino acid profile is often less aligned with human tissue needs, and the food matrix may reduce digestibility or dilute the protein inside a larger burden of fiber, starch, and antinutrient chemistry. The result is that more total food, more total calories, or more strategic combining may be needed just to approximate the leucine-driven signal a smaller serving of animal protein can provide more directly.

Age makes the threshold problem even sharper. As people get older, muscle becomes less responsive to weak protein signals, a pattern often described as anabolic resistance. The machinery still works, but it takes a stronger amino acid and leucine stimulus to turn it on effectively. This is one reason why light, low-protein meals that appear reasonable on paper can quietly fail older adults. They may preserve appetite just enough to look adequate while underdelivering the signal needed to maintain lean tissue. Over time that matters. Muscle mass is not only about strength or appearance. It affects metabolic stability, glucose disposal, resilience during illness, balance, recovery, and survival itself. If meals repeatedly miss the leucine threshold, the body spends more time in turnover than in rebuilding.

This is why muscle maintenance depends on more than hitting a daily protein total in the abstract. The meal has to be built strongly enough to trigger synthesis when it arrives. That means enough digestible protein, enough leucine, and enough overall essential amino acid support to make the signal real. Otherwise the body receives fragments of instruction rather than a full directive to repair and maintain tissue. Leucine threshold is therefore not a niche bodybuilding concept. It is one of the clearest examples of how food quality, digestibility, and amino acid pattern determine whether protein becomes real structure or remains a partially wasted opportunity.

Aging, Anabolic Resistance, and Protein Efficiency

Aging changes protein metabolism by making the body harder to convince. The machinery for building and repairing tissue does not disappear, but it becomes less responsive to weak nutritional signals. This is what anabolic resistance means. Anabolism is the building side of metabolism, the side that assembles new protein into muscle, connective tissue, enzymes, and repair structures. Resistance means the signal that once would have triggered a strong synthetic response now produces a smaller one. The older body often needs a denser protein input, a stronger essential amino acid rise, and a more decisive leucine signal before muscle protein synthesis turns on meaningfully. That shift matters because aging does not reduce the need for repair. It increases it. Protein turnover continues. Muscle fibers still experience wear. Connective tissues still need maintenance. Immune demand does not disappear. The body is still trying to rebuild itself, but the nutritional threshold required to drive that rebuilding has moved upward.

This is why light, diluted, or low-quality protein intake becomes more costly with age. A younger person may be able to coast longer on mediocre protein distribution, low-protein breakfasts, or plant-heavy meals with weaker amino acid density and still preserve acceptable lean mass for a while. The older organism loses that margin. A meal that looks reasonable on paper may fail to deliver enough digestible essential amino acids to cross the anabolic threshold. The person may eat, feel fed, and still fail to generate a strong repair response in muscle and other tissues. This is how aging and protein insufficiency often hide inside ordinary eating patterns. The diet does not have to look extreme. It only has to become too weak relative to the body's rising threshold for synthesis. Over time, missed signals accumulate as reduced lean mass, slower recovery, lower strength, poorer balance, reduced metabolic flexibility, and greater vulnerability during illness or injury.

Protein efficiency becomes critical in that setting because the question is no longer merely how much protein is present in the meal. The question is how much of that protein digestion can actually liberate, how complete the amino acid pattern is, how much leucine is delivered, and how much food volume or digestive work the body has to spend in order to get there. Animal proteins tend to perform well because they are dense, highly digestible, and rich in the essential amino acids needed to drive synthesis. Once stomach acid, pancreatic proteases, and brush-border enzymes have done their work, the bloodstream sees a sharper and more useful amino acid rise. Many lower-quality protein sources are less efficient because they provide a weaker essential amino acid pattern, less leucine per serving, more dilution by fiber or carbohydrate, or more digestive interference from plant defense chemistry. In an older body, those inefficiencies matter more. The margin for soft signals is smaller.

The cost of ignoring this is not confined to muscle aesthetics. Lean tissue is part of metabolic stability itself. Muscle acts as a major site of glucose disposal. It helps maintain physical capacity, supports resilience under stress, and provides a reserve the body can draw on during infection, trauma, or reduced intake. When anabolic resistance meets poor protein efficiency, the body begins living on thinner structural margins. Recovery after exertion becomes less complete. Small losses in lean tissue become harder to reverse. Illness becomes more expensive because the body has less amino acid-rich tissue to spare and less dietary efficiency coming in to replace what is lost. A person can remain overfed in calories and under-supported in protein-driven repair at the same time. Aging makes that mismatch more dangerous, not less.

This is why protein quality and meal construction matter more as the body gets older. The goal is not simply to consume protein somewhere in the day and hope total intake averages out. The goal is to deliver enough high-quality, digestible protein in individual meals to overcome anabolic resistance and produce a real synthetic response. That means stronger amino acid density, stronger leucine delivery, and less reliance on foods that force the body to work harder for a weaker return. Aging narrows the space for nutritional vagueness. The body becomes less forgiving of diluted protein and more dependent on efficient protein biology. Protein efficiency is therefore not a performance luxury for the elderly. It is part of preserving structure in a system that no longer responds well to weak signals.

Why Digestibility Changes the Real Value of Food Protein

Protein is only valuable to the body to the extent that digestion can turn it into absorbable amino acids and small peptides. That is the first correction. Food protein is not useful merely because laboratory analysis detects nitrogen-containing compounds in the product. Until stomach acid denatures those proteins, until pepsin and pancreatic proteases cut them down, until brush-border enzymes finish the last trimming work at the intestinal surface, and until the resulting amino acids cross into the bloodstream, the body does not yet have the protein it appears to have eaten. This is why digestibility changes everything. It determines whether the protein listed on paper becomes structural material in circulation or remains partly trapped inside food matrix, passes through incompletely processed, or reaches the colon as residue instead of nourishment.

Animal protein usually performs well because the digestive system can dismantle it with relatively high efficiency. The proteins are complete, the amino acid pattern aligns closely with human needs, and once acid and proteases have done their work the intestine can extract a large share of what was present. The body spends digestive effort and gets a strong return. Many plant proteins behave differently. They may be diluted by fiber, locked inside cell structures, or paired with protease inhibitors, lectins, tannins, and other compounds that reduce the efficiency of breakdown and absorption. So the issue is not only that the amino acid profile may be weaker. The issue is that the body may physically recover less of the protein that was there to begin with. The food can still be called high protein. The tissues may still receive far less usable amino acid material than the label implies.

This is where digestibility and protein quality start to merge. A food with a strong amino acid profile but poor digestibility loses real value because too little of that profile reaches the bloodstream intact. A food with a weaker amino acid profile and poor digestibility loses twice. First in composition, then again in extraction. This is why equal grams of protein from different foods are not equal biological events. One meal may yield a sharp rise in circulating essential amino acids, including enough leucine to support muscle protein synthesis and broader tissue repair. Another may require more total food volume, more total calories, and more digestive effort just to generate a weaker amino acid rise that still fails to cross the threshold for optimal synthesis. The protein number survives on the label. The protein effect shrinks in the body.

Digestibility matters even more when digestive function is compromised. Low stomach acid, weak pancreatic output, damaged brush-border function, intestinal inflammation, rushed eating, or poor meal context can all reduce the body's ability to extract amino acids cleanly. A protein source that is only marginally digestible under ideal conditions becomes even less valuable when the digestive sequence is under strain. That is one reason people can believe they are eating enough protein while still showing the consequences of underdelivery. Recovery weakens. Lean mass becomes harder to maintain. Satiety becomes less reliable. Hair, skin, connective tissue, and immune resilience begin to show the cost. The diet may be adequate by arithmetic and inadequate by physiology.

This is why digestibility changes the real value of food protein. The body does not build itself from theoretical protein. It builds itself from amino acids that were actually liberated, absorbed, transported, and used. A food deserves to be called a good protein source only if digestion can turn it into that reality with a high enough yield. Protein on paper is composition. Digestible protein is nourishment.

Part IV

Fat as Structure, Fuel, and Signal

Chapter 13

Why Fat Digestion Is Different

Fat does not mix with water because fat molecules and water molecules are built around different chemical priorities. Water is polar. Its electrical charge is distributed unevenly, which makes water molecules strongly attracted to one another and to other charged or polar substances. Fat is largely nonpolar. The long hydrocarbon chains that make up fatty acids do not carry that same uneven charge pattern, so they do not interact comfortably with water. When fat enters an aqueous environment such as the stomach contents or the small intestine, it does not dissolve into the surrounding fluid the way salt or sugar can. It pulls away, gathers into droplets, and minimizes contact with water. This is not a minor culinary detail. It is the first major physical problem of fat digestion. The intestine is a water-based space. Digestive enzymes are operating in fluid. Blood and lymph are fluid transport systems. If dietary fat remains clustered in large globules, the body cannot access it efficiently.

That clustering matters because enzymes work at surfaces. Pancreatic lipase does not magically penetrate an intact mass of oil or melted fat and digest it from the inside out. It has to bind at the interface between fat and the watery digestive environment. A large fat droplet has relatively little surface area compared with its volume, which means only a small fraction of the total fat is accessible at any one time. The bigger the droplet, the worse the access problem becomes. Protein digestion is different because protein can be denatured by acid and cleaved by proteases directly in solution or suspension. Carbohydrate digestion is different because sugars and starch breakdown products are far more compatible with water. Fat resists that entire logic. It separates from the medium in which digestion is taking place. The body therefore cannot treat fat like another soluble nutrient. It has to change fat's physical presentation first.

This is why bile is indispensable. The liver makes bile acids, and the gallbladder stores and concentrates them for release when fat reaches the small intestine. Bile acids have a split chemical personality. Part of the molecule interacts with water. Another part interacts with fat. That allows bile acids to surround fat droplets and break large masses into much smaller ones, a process called emulsification. Emulsification does not digest the fat yet. It makes digestion possible. It increases the total surface area exposed to pancreatic lipase and creates microscopic lipid particles that the rest of the digestive system can actually work with. Without this step, large amounts of dietary fat would remain chemically present and biologically inaccessible. The food could be rich in lipid energy and fat-soluble vitamins, and the body would still struggle to extract them because the physical format was wrong.

So when it is said that fat does not mix with water, the real meaning is deeper than kitchen observation. It means dietary fat enters the gut as a structural problem that the body has to solve before absorption can begin. The organism needs fats for membranes, hormones, long-duration fuel, and transport of fat-soluble vitamins, but first it has to overcome the fact that fat naturally resists the medium in which digestion occurs. That is why fat digestion is different from the start. It begins not with simple cleavage, but with separation, emulsification, and controlled access.

Why Bile Physiology Is Central to Fat Digestion

Bile physiology is central to fat digestion because fat cannot be handled efficiently by the digestive tract until its physical form has been changed. Protein can be denatured by acid and cut by proteases. Carbohydrate can be hydrolyzed into sugars that move easily through the watery environment of the intestine. Fat behaves differently from the beginning. It separates, gathers, and resists contact with the fluid medium where digestion is taking place. That makes bile indispensable. Without bile, dietary fat remains present but poorly accessible. The meal can contain enormous lipid energy, fat-soluble vitamins, phospholipids, and cholesterol, yet the body still cannot reach them cleanly because the physical presentation of the fat is wrong for enzyme access. Bile is what solves that problem. It is the system that turns fat from a clustered, water-repelling mass into something the intestine can actually work on.

The chemistry of bile explains why. Bile acids are made from cholesterol in the liver and released into the intestine when dietary fat arrives. Their structure is amphipathic, meaning one side of the molecule interacts with water while the other side interacts with fat. That split character allows bile acids to surround large lipid droplets and disperse them into much smaller ones. This is emulsification. The fat has not yet been digested, but the total surface area exposed to pancreatic lipase has expanded dramatically. That matters because lipase acts only at the lipid-water interface. The larger the interface, the more effectively the enzyme can hydrolyze triglycerides into fatty acids and monoglycerides. So bile is not optional support around the edges of fat digestion. It creates the physical condition that makes meaningful fat digestion possible in the first place.

Bile physiology is also central because the job does not end with emulsification. Once lipase has begun breaking fat down, the intestine still has to move those digestion products through an aqueous lumen to the absorptive surface. Free fatty acids, monoglycerides, cholesterol, and fat-soluble vitamins do not travel well in water on their own. Bile acids organize them into micelles, small transport assemblies that carry these hydrophobic molecules through the intestinal fluid and bring them into contact with the brush border of the enterocyte, the absorptive cell lining the intestine. Without micelle formation, even hydrolyzed fat would remain poorly delivered. The digestive system would have broken the lipid apart chemically while still failing to move it efficiently to the site of absorption. Bile therefore sits at both stages of the problem. It first makes fat accessible to enzymes. Then it makes the products of that digestion deliverable to the membrane.

This is why bile problems show up as much more than vague fat intolerance. If bile production is weak, if gallbladder release is poor, if bile flow is obstructed, or if the bile acid pool is impaired, fat digestion becomes less efficient and fat absorption falls with it. The person may notice greasy stools, bloating, heaviness after fatty meals, poor tolerance for richer foods, or a general sense that fat just sits there. But the deeper issue is nutritional. Fat-soluble vitamins A, D, E, and K depend on this same bile-mediated system for absorption. Cholesterol handling changes. Satiety from fat-rich meals may weaken because the digestion is incomplete. The body may receive less of the very lipid material it uses for membranes, steroid hormone synthesis, nervous system function, and long-duration fuel. In other words, poor bile physiology does not simply reduce comfort. It lowers access to an entire class of structurally and metabolically important nutrients.

The timing of bile release makes the point even sharper. The liver produces bile continuously, but the gallbladder stores and concentrates it so a strong pulse can be delivered when fat enters the duodenum. That coordination shows how seriously the body treats fat digestion. It does not leak a little detergent into the gut and hope for the best. It prepares, stores, and releases a concentrated solution at the right moment because fat digestion requires a properly timed physical intervention before chemical digestion and absorption can proceed. Bile physiology is therefore not a side detail in nutrition. It is one of the core reasons dietary fat can become usable biology instead of remaining partly stranded in the lumen as inaccessible energy.

Why Fat Digestion Depends on Coordination, Not Just One Enzyme

Fat digestion is often described too simply, as if pancreatic lipase were the star of the process and everything else were background support. That picture is wrong because lipase cannot solve the basic problem of dietary fat by itself. Fat reaches the intestine as a hydrophobic mass that resists the watery environment where digestion has to occur. Before any enzyme can work well, the meal has to be recognized, gastric emptying has to be timed, bile has to be produced by the liver and released by the gallbladder, acid leaving the stomach has to be neutralized, fat droplets have to be emulsified, and the intestinal environment has to be physically organized so lipase can even reach the substrate. Then, after lipase has done its cutting, the products still have to be packaged into micelles, delivered to the absorptive surface, taken into enterocytes, reassembled into triglycerides, packed into chylomicrons, and sent through lymphatic transport. This is not a one-enzyme story. It is a coordinated sequence of mechanical timing, chemical restructuring, enzymatic hydrolysis, membrane transfer, and transport logistics.

The coordination begins before the small intestine ever sees the meal. Fat in the stomach slows gastric emptying, which changes how quickly chyme is delivered downstream. That delay is not an inconvenience. It is part of the design. The small intestine needs time to prepare for a more complex digestive event than simple carbohydrate handling. When fat reaches the duodenum, intestinal cells release cholecystokinin, or CCK, a hormone that signals the gallbladder to contract and the pancreas to release digestive secretions. At the same time, pancreatic bicarbonate helps neutralize the acidity of chyme arriving from the stomach, because the enzymes that digest fat do not work properly in the highly acidic environment the stomach uses for protein denaturation. Already the pattern is clear. Before lipase can do meaningful work, hormone signaling, biliary release, and pH control all have to line up correctly.

Bile is the next major requirement, and it proves the same point. Lipase works at the surface of fat droplets. If those droplets remain large, surface area stays small and enzymatic access remains poor. Bile acids solve that physical problem by emulsifying fat into much smaller droplets, creating a vastly larger working surface. But even here lipase is not enough on its own. Bile acids are necessary for access, yet the same bile environment can interfere with how lipase sits on the fat droplet unless colipase is present to stabilize that interaction. So the system already requires multiple coordinated players even at the level of direct enzymatic attack. Bile makes fat reachable. Colipase helps lipase stay engaged. Lipase then hydrolyzes triglycerides into fatty acids and monoglycerides. Remove any one of those pieces and the whole process weakens.

Absorption adds another layer of dependency. Even after triglycerides have been cut apart, the resulting lipid fragments do not simply dissolve and drift into the bloodstream. They still have to move through an aqueous lumen, which means bile acids must help organize them into micelles so they can be delivered to the brush border of the intestinal cell. Once inside the enterocyte, the lipid fragments are re-esterified, meaning rebuilt into triglycerides, then packaged with cholesterol, phospholipids, and apolipoproteins into chylomicrons. Those particles are too large to move directly into the capillaries that handle amino acids and sugars, so they enter the lymphatic system first. In other words, even perfect lipase activity would not finish the job without intact micelle formation, enterocyte function, intracellular repackaging, and lymphatic transport. Fat digestion depends on a chain. A chain is only as strong as its weakest step.

This is why people can have trouble with fat digestion for reasons that have nothing to do with "not enough enzyme" in isolation. The issue may be poor bile flow, impaired gallbladder contraction, weak hormonal signaling, inadequate bicarbonate buffering, damaged intestinal absorption, poor chylomicron assembly, or multiple smaller defects acting together. The body may respond with bloating, heaviness after fatty meals, pale or greasy stools, poor tolerance for richer foods, or reduced absorption of fat-soluble vitamins. Those symptoms are the visible edge of a coordination failure. Fat digestion is not a single chemical cut. It is a tightly timed system that turns water-repelling dietary lipid into absorbable, transportable biological material. That is why it depends on coordination, not just one enzyme.

Why Digestion Changes When Fat Becomes a Major Energy Source

When fat becomes a major energy source, the digestive system is not dealing with a small supporting nutrient anymore. It is being asked to process a larger share of the meal through bile-dependent, lipase-dependent, slower-moving pathways rather than through rapid glucose handling. That changes the entire rhythm of digestion. Fat delays gastric emptying, increases the need for coordinated bile release, raises dependence on pancreatic lipase and colipase, and shifts more of the absorptive workload toward micelle formation, enterocyte repackaging, and lymphatic transport. A diet built around frequent refined carbohydrate asks the gut to move fast and the pancreas to contain repeated glucose entry. A diet built around larger amounts of fat asks the gut to slow down, emulsify carefully, hydrolyze thoroughly, and distribute fuel over a longer period. The difference is not philosophical. It is anatomical and chemical. The same organs are involved, but the balance of their work changes.

The gallbladder becomes especially important under those conditions because bile has to be delivered reliably and in sufficient concentration to handle the incoming fat load. The liver is always producing bile, but when dietary fat becomes a central fuel source, the demand for timed bile release becomes more frequent and more consequential. If bile flow is weak, if gallbladder contraction is sluggish, or if the body has spent years on a lower-fat pattern and is not yet handling richer meals smoothly, the transition can feel heavy. The person may notice fullness, bloating, pale or greasy stools, loose stools, or a sense that richer food does not sit cleanly. This does not prove that fat is inherently wrong for the person. Often it means the mechanical side of fat digestion has not fully adapted to the new workload yet. The chemistry is asking for stronger biliary coordination than the system has been using recently.

The small intestine also changes its role because a larger share of nutrient extraction now depends on emulsification and micelle-mediated transport rather than fast carbohydrate absorption. Fat digestion is slower because the body has to solve more steps before it can claim the energy. Large droplets have to be broken into small ones. Triglycerides have to be hydrolyzed into fatty acids and monoglycerides. Those products have to be brought to the absorptive surface, taken into enterocytes, rebuilt into triglycerides, and packaged into chylomicrons before they enter lymphatic circulation. That longer route is exactly why fat tends to provide steadier post-meal energy and stronger satiety when digestion is functioning well. The fuel enters more gradually. The body is not being flooded with rapid glucose that has to be contained immediately through insulin. Instead, energy arrives through a slower and more extended stream that can support a more stable metabolic state.

Hormonal signaling changes with it. Meals richer in fat and protein stimulate cholecystokinin more strongly, slow gastric emptying, and often suppress appetite for longer because the meal is still being processed and meaningful structural material is still entering circulation. The endocrine message becomes different from that produced by frequent refined carbohydrate intake. Less rapid glucose entry often means less repeated insulin pressure and more reliance on fat oxidation between meals. That shift can feel unfamiliar at first because the person is moving from a metabolism trained around repeated short-interval fuel delivery to one that is being asked to tolerate longer, steadier access to energy. During that change, the digestive system and the broader metabolic system are adapting together. Bile handling, pancreatic output, gastric pacing, satiety signaling, and cellular fuel preference are all being asked to operate in a different pattern.

This is why digestion changes when fat becomes a major energy source. The body is not just eating more of the same thing. It is reweighting the digestive sequence toward a slower, more coordinated, more bile-centered form of nutrient handling. When that system is working well, the result is often stronger satiety, steadier energy, and less dependence on constant feeding. When it is underprepared, the person may temporarily experience fat as difficult. The correct conclusion is not simply that fat is the problem. The better question is whether the digestive architecture responsible for fat handling, liver, gallbladder, pancreas, intestinal absorption, and lymphatic transport, is meeting the new workload cleanly enough to make that fuel available.

Chapter 14

The Liver, Gallbladder, and Bile System

Bile begins in the liver because fat digestion has to be prepared before fat ever reaches the absorptive surface of the intestine. The liver does not wait for a meal and then improvise. It manufactures bile continuously, building the chemical tool the body will later use to make dietary fat accessible. This alone says something important about human physiology. Fat digestion is not a side pathway or a backup trick. The organism invests permanent liver tissue, permanent synthetic capacity, and permanent transport architecture into producing the fluid required to handle lipids well. That fluid is bile, and its central active components are bile acids, molecules made from cholesterol inside hepatocytes, the main working cells of the liver. Cholesterol is not merely circulating debris to be discussed on a lab report. Part of its biological destiny is to be turned into bile acids so the body can digest and absorb fat at all.

The chemistry matters because bile acids solve a physical problem the rest of digestion cannot solve cleanly. Fat does not dissolve into the aqueous environment of the intestine. It separates, gathers, and resists contact with the watery medium where enzymes operate. Bile acids are built with two different faces. One side interacts with water. The other side interacts with fat. That amphipathic structure is what gives them detergent-like behavior. The liver takes cholesterol, modifies it through a sequence of enzymatic reactions, and produces bile acids that can later surround lipid droplets and break their large masses into smaller dispersed particles. This is emulsification. It is not yet fat digestion in the narrow sense, because triglycerides have not been hydrolyzed by lipase at that stage, but it is the prerequisite that makes meaningful lipase access possible. The liver is therefore producing not just a secretion, but the chemical condition that allows fat digestion to happen efficiently downstream.

Bile is more than bile acids alone. The liver also places phospholipids, cholesterol, bilirubin, electrolytes, and water into the bile stream. Phospholipids support the organization of lipids in solution. Cholesterol is carried in bile both as part of normal lipid handling and as one route by which the body disposes of excess cholesterol. Bilirubin, a pigment derived from the breakdown of heme, the iron-containing component of hemoglobin, enters bile as part of waste processing. This means bile production sits at the intersection of digestion and disposal. The same fluid that later helps absorb fats and fat-soluble vitamins also carries waste products the body intends to eliminate through the intestine. The liver is doing both jobs at once. It is preparing a digestive tool and packaging chemical waste into the same outgoing stream.

That stream begins inside the microscopic architecture of the liver. Hepatocytes secrete bile into tiny channels called canaliculi, and those channels collect bile into progressively larger ducts. From there the fluid moves through the biliary tree toward the common hepatic duct, where it can either flow onward toward the intestine or be diverted into the gallbladder for storage and concentration. This means bile production is continuous even when no meal is being eaten. The liver keeps generating the fluid because the body cannot afford to start from zero the moment dietary fat appears. A high-fat meal would outpace the system if bile had to be built from scratch each time. Continuous production solves that problem. The gallbladder then adds timing and concentration later, but the chemical work begins in the liver.

This is why liver health matters so much in fat digestion. A liver that is overburdened, inflamed, infiltrated with excess fat, or impaired in bile synthesis does not just create a laboratory abnormality. It changes what the intestine will later be able to do with dietary fat. Poor bile production means weaker emulsification, weaker micelle formation, and weaker absorption of fatty acids, cholesterol, and fat-soluble vitamins such as vitamins A, D, E, and K. A person may then interpret the result as poor tolerance for fat, when part of the real problem is that the liver is not supplying the chemical machinery required to process that fat cleanly. The meal may be correct in principle. The upstream preparation may be inadequate.

Bile production in the liver is therefore not a minor supporting detail in nutrition. It is one of the clearest examples of how the body invests real organ function into making a certain class of nutrients usable. The liver takes cholesterol, builds bile acids, packages them into bile, and sends that fluid into the biliary system so fat can later be emulsified, absorbed, and turned into fuel, membrane material, and hormonal substrate. Before the intestine can claim lipid nutrition, the liver has already gone to work.

Gallbladder Storage and Timed Release

The gallbladder exists because bile production and bile use do not occur on the same schedule. The liver makes bile continuously, but the intestine does not need a steady trickle of bile at all times. It needs a concentrated release at the moment dietary fat actually arrives. That is the gallbladder's role. It stores bile between meals, concentrates it by removing water and certain electrolytes, and then delivers it in a timed pulse when fat enters the duodenum, the first section of the small intestine. Without that timing system, the body would still have bile, but it would not have the same force of delivery. The chemistry would exist in the wrong distribution. Fat digestion would become less efficient because the intestine would receive too little bile when the real workload appeared.

This is not a passive storage job. The gallbladder changes bile while it holds it. As water is reabsorbed, bile acids, phospholipids, cholesterol, and pigments become more concentrated. That matters because fat digestion depends on enough emulsifying power being present at once to break large lipid masses into smaller droplets with dramatically increased surface area. A diluted bile stream would do the same kind of work more weakly. The gallbladder solves that by turning continuous liver output into a more potent digestive release. It is effectively a pressure system for lipid handling. The liver supplies the chemistry. The gallbladder supplies concentration and timing.

The timing itself is controlled hormonally. When fat reaches the small intestine, cells in the intestinal lining release cholecystokinin, or CCK. That hormone travels through blood and signals the gallbladder to contract. At the same time, it helps relax the sphincter of Oddi, the muscular gate that regulates flow from the bile duct and pancreatic duct into the intestine. This coordination matters because bile and pancreatic enzymes need access to the same meal at the same time. Emulsification and lipase activity are linked. If the gallbladder contracts weakly, too late, or against a poorly relaxed outlet, the meal can enter a phase of impaired fat handling even when the liver is making bile normally. The chemistry exists. The delivery fails.

This is why gallbladder function shapes how a person experiences richer meals. When storage and release are working properly, dietary fat enters the intestine, bile is released in a concentrated burst, emulsification proceeds efficiently, pancreatic lipase gains access to the lipid surface, and fat digestion can move forward with relatively little friction. When that coordination is poor, the person may notice heaviness, bloating, nausea, upper abdominal discomfort, pale or greasy stools, or a sense that fatty meals sit badly. Those symptoms are not always about the fat itself. Often they are about timing failure. The meal arrived. The bile pulse did not match it well enough.

The gallbladder therefore makes a broader point about human digestion. Nutrients are not handled just by chemical presence. They are handled by timing, concentration, sequencing, and organ coordination. The body does not merely need bile somewhere in the system. It needs bile in the right place, in the right amount, at the right moment. That is what the gallbladder provides. It turns continuous hepatic production into targeted digestive force, and in doing so it makes fat digestion cleaner, faster, and more effective than liver output alone could manage.

Emulsification and Microscopic Fat Dispersion

Emulsification is the step where the body solves the physical problem of fat before it can solve the chemical one. Dietary fat does not arrive in the intestine as a fine, easily digested mist. It arrives as larger hydrophobic masses that pull away from the surrounding water-based digestive fluid. Left alone, those masses offer very little usable surface for enzyme attack. Pancreatic lipase cannot meaningfully digest the interior of a large fat droplet. It works at the interface, the boundary where fat meets water. That means the body has to change the geometry of the meal before fat digestion can proceed efficiently. It has to take a relatively small number of larger lipid globules and turn them into an enormous number of much smaller droplets. The chemistry of the fat has not changed yet. The physical presentation has. That change is emulsification, and it is one of the most important mechanical events in digestion.

Bile acids make it possible because they are built with two different loyalties. One side of the molecule interacts with water. The other side interacts with fat. When bile enters the small intestine and encounters a lipid mass, these molecules position themselves at the fat-water boundary and begin breaking the larger globule apart into smaller droplets. This is not random breakup. It is controlled stabilization. As the droplets become smaller, bile acids coat their surface and help prevent them from simply merging back into one larger mass. The result is microscopic fat dispersion, a far wider distribution of tiny lipid particles suspended through the intestinal contents rather than a few large resistant pools of oil and melted fat. The body has not digested the fat yet, but it has turned the meal into something digestive enzymes can finally approach with real efficiency.

The importance of size here is not cosmetic. It is mathematical. A single large droplet contains a huge amount of fat but exposes relatively little total surface area. Break that same mass into thousands of microscopic droplets and the total exposed surface rises dramatically. That larger collective surface is exactly what pancreatic lipase needs. The enzyme now has access to far more triglyceride boundary and can begin hydrolyzing the fat into free fatty acids and monoglycerides at a much faster and more complete rate. Without microscopic dispersion, the enzyme is functionally starved of access even though the fat is physically present in the lumen. This is one of the central lessons of digestion. Presence is not access. A nutrient can be sitting in the gut and still remain partly unavailable until the body changes its physical form.

Emulsification also prepares the way for the next transport problem. Once lipase begins cutting triglycerides apart, the resulting lipid fragments still do not move comfortably through the aqueous intestinal environment on their own. The same bile system that created microscopic droplets now helps organize those digestion products into micellar structures, tiny transport assemblies that carry fatty acids, monoglycerides, cholesterol, and fat-soluble vitamins through the intestinal fluid to the absorptive surface. So emulsification is not an isolated trick. It is the opening move in a longer sequence that runs from fat dispersion to enzymatic hydrolysis to micelle delivery to intestinal absorption. If the first step is weak, the rest of the chain weakens with it.

This is why poor emulsification can quietly lower the value of an otherwise nutrient-dense meal. The food may contain substantial fat energy, phospholipids, cholesterol, and vitamins A, D, E, and K, but if bile delivery is poor or microscopic dispersion is incomplete, the body may extract much less than the meal appears to offer. The label can remain impressive while the intestine receives a thinner return. Emulsification and microscopic fat dispersion are therefore not side details in fat digestion. They are the point where the body turns a water-repelling mass into a digestible and eventually absorbable nutrient stream.

Enterohepatic Recycling

Bile is too valuable for the body to use once and discard carelessly. That is why most bile acids are not lost after they help digest a meal. They are recovered, returned to the liver, and used again through a circulation loop called enterohepatic recycling. The term sounds technical, but the logic is simple. Entero refers to the intestine. Hepatic refers to the liver. Recycling means the body is pulling bile acids back out of the intestinal stream after they have done their work and routing them upstream for reuse. This is not a minor efficiency trick. It is one of the reasons the body can digest fat meal after meal without having to synthesize a completely new bile acid supply every time.

The sequence begins in the liver, where bile acids are made from cholesterol and secreted into bile. The gallbladder stores and concentrates that bile between meals, then releases it into the duodenum when fat enters the small intestine. There, bile acids emulsify fat, help create microscopic lipid droplets, and later organize digestion products into micelles so fatty acids, monoglycerides, cholesterol, and fat-soluble vitamins can be brought to the absorptive surface of the intestine. Once that job is mostly finished, the bile acids themselves are still in the intestinal lumen. If the body simply discarded them all in stool, it would need to replace a large amount of bile chemistry constantly. That would be metabolically expensive and would increase the need for fresh cholesterol conversion in the liver just to keep up.

Instead, the body reclaims most of them in the terminal ileum, the final section of the small intestine. Specialized transport systems in the ileal lining pull bile acids back across the intestinal membrane and return them to portal blood, the venous system that carries absorbed material directly to the liver. From there the liver takes them back up, resecretes them into bile, and sends them out again for future meals. This loop can run repeatedly. A single bile acid molecule may participate in digestion many times before it is eventually lost. The liver does still synthesize new bile acids, because some are always excreted and have to be replaced, but the majority are conserved through this cycle rather than constantly rebuilt from scratch.

That conservation matters because fat digestion depends on having enough bile acids available at the right moment. If the bile acid pool falls, the intestine loses emulsifying power and micelle formation weakens. Fat can remain less accessible to lipase, and fat-soluble vitamins can become harder to absorb. So enterohepatic recycling is not just about efficiency. It protects digestive competence. It preserves the chemical tools needed for repeated lipid handling and keeps fat digestion from becoming unnecessarily fragile. A system built to use fat as a meaningful nutrient and fuel source cannot afford to waste its detergent chemistry every time a meal is eaten.

This also means that disruption anywhere in the loop can create downstream problems. Poor bile production in the liver, weak gallbladder release, damage to the ileum, or altered intestinal conditions that impair bile acid recovery can all reduce the effective bile acid pool. The result may show up as poor fat tolerance, greasy stools, bloating after fatty meals, or weaker absorption of vitamins A, D, E, and K. In that sense, enterohepatic recycling is one of the clearest examples of how digestion is not a straight line from mouth to stool. It is a managed circulation system in which the body repeatedly reclaims what it needs, reuses what is expensive to make, and keeps the chemistry of nourishment running through conservation as well as secretion.

What Poor Bile Flow Does to Digestion and Nutrient Absorption

Poor bile flow weakens fat digestion at the first physical step, which means the body can be eating fat, fat-soluble vitamins, cholesterol, and phospholipids without extracting them cleanly. The problem begins before absorption. Dietary fat enters the small intestine as larger hydrophobic masses that do not mix with the watery intestinal environment. Bile acids are supposed to solve that by coating those lipid masses, breaking them into much smaller droplets, and creating the surface area pancreatic lipase needs in order to hydrolyze triglycerides into fatty acids and monoglycerides. When bile flow is poor, that dispersion step weakens. Larger droplets remain. Enzyme access falls. Fat stays present in the lumen but less of it becomes digestible substrate. This is one of the clearest examples of why presence is not access. The meal may contain rich lipid nutrition. The intestine may still be left with poor extraction.

That failure then spreads downstream. If emulsification is incomplete, micelle formation is weaker as well. Micelles are the small transport assemblies that carry fatty acids, monoglycerides, cholesterol, and fat-soluble vitamins through the aqueous intestinal contents to the absorptive surface of the enterocyte, the absorptive cell lining the intestine. Without enough bile acids moving through the system, those lipid digestion products are delivered less efficiently to the membrane. So poor bile flow does not simply make the first stage of fat handling slower. It lowers the entire chain of access from droplet dispersion to enzyme action to membrane delivery. The result is that less dietary fat crosses into the body in usable form, even when the person is eating enough.

Fat-soluble vitamins are often where this shows up nutritionally. Vitamins A, D, E, and K ride with fat digestion. If bile flow is poor, their absorption can fall along with fat itself because they depend on the same micellar transport system to reach the intestinal surface. This means a person can eat foods that contain these vitamins and still develop a thinner effective supply at the tissue level. The same meal that should have delivered membrane-supporting fats, hormone-building substrate, and fat-soluble vitamins becomes a lower-yield event because the chemical machinery needed to carry those compounds inward was underpowered. The label can remain impressive. The body receives less.

The digestive symptoms often reflect this chemistry directly. Fat that is not properly emulsified and absorbed remains in the intestinal contents and moves further down the tract than it should. The person may notice heaviness after richer meals, bloating, nausea, a sense that fat sits in the gut, pale stools, loose stools, floating stools, or greasy residue in the stool because unabsorbed lipid is being carried out instead of claimed. That is not merely discomfort. It is evidence of lost nutrient extraction. The colon is then forced to deal with material that should have been handled and absorbed much earlier. The meal becomes residue instead of nourishment.

Poor bile flow also changes satiety and energy in quieter ways. Fat-rich meals normally slow gastric emptying, create a longer digestive timeline, and help support steadier post-meal energy because lipid absorption unfolds more gradually than rapid glucose absorption. If bile flow is weak, that same meal may feel heavy without producing the same clean satiety. The digestive system senses the fat load, but extraction is less efficient and the nutritional return is lower. The person may leave the meal feeling full and unsatisfied at the same time, burdened mechanically but underfed chemically. That mismatch is common whenever digestion imposes work that is not matched by good yield.

This is why bile flow matters far beyond gallbladder comfort or occasional intolerance to rich food. It determines whether a major class of nutrients can be made available to the organism at all. Poor bile flow means weaker emulsification, weaker micelle formation, weaker lipid absorption, weaker fat-soluble vitamin delivery, more residue in the gut, and a lower real value from foods that should have been dense nutritional inputs. The body can only use the fats and lipid-soluble compounds that bile helps make accessible. When that flow is poor, the meal does not disappear. It simply feeds the organism less effectively while burdening the intestine more.

Chapter 15

Fat Absorption, Lymphatic Transport, and Stable Energy

Once bile has dispersed dietary fat into microscopic droplets, the next major step is chemical cleavage, and that step belongs largely to pancreatic lipase. Most of the fat people eat arrives as triglyceride, a molecule built from three fatty acids attached to a glycerol backbone. In that intact form, the molecule is energy-dense but not yet absorbable. The intestine cannot simply pull whole triglycerides across the membrane and call the job done. The fatty acids have to be freed from the backbone first, at least in large part, so the digestion products can be organized into micelles, carried to the absorptive surface, and taken into enterocytes, the absorptive cells lining the small intestine. Pancreatic lipase performs that cut. It hydrolyzes triglycerides mainly at the first and third positions on the glycerol backbone, releasing two free fatty acids and leaving behind a 2-monoglyceride, a glycerol molecule still holding one fatty acid in the middle position. That combination, free fatty acids and monoglycerides, is the main output of efficient triglyceride digestion.

This process depends on access as much as chemistry. Lipase is an enzyme that works at the lipid-water boundary, not deep inside a large mass of oil. That is why bile has to act first. Emulsification creates the surface. Lipase then attacks that surface. Even here the body uses another layer of coordination, because bile acids, while necessary for dispersion, can also interfere with how lipase sits on the droplet. Colipase solves that problem. It acts as an anchoring partner, helping lipase bind effectively to the emulsified fat surface so hydrolysis can proceed. The body is therefore not throwing one enzyme at the meal and hoping for the best. It is staging the event carefully. Bile creates access. Colipase stabilizes the working position. Lipase cuts. Only then do the major products of triglyceride digestion become available for transport.

The importance of this step is easy to underestimate because fat digestion is often discussed as if absorption simply follows automatically once the meal enters the small intestine. It does not. Until triglycerides are broken into smaller lipid units, the intestine has little to work with. The fatty acids remain trapped inside a larger storage molecule whose structure is excellent for biological energy storage but poor for direct membrane transfer. Lipase changes that by turning packed energy into transportable fragments. Those fragments can then join bile-acid micelles, move through the aqueous intestinal lumen, and approach the brush border where absorption becomes possible. In other words, pancreatic lipase does not finish fat digestion by itself, but it performs the decisive cut that turns dietary triglyceride from stored chemistry into absorbable lipid material.

This is why poor lipase activity changes so much downstream. If lipase output is weak, if the pancreatic contribution to digestion is impaired, or if bile-mediated access is poor enough that lipase cannot engage properly, fat may stay partly intact and move further down the intestine than it should. The person may feel heavy after rich meals, notice greasy stool, or fail to absorb lipid nutrients cleanly even while eating enough fat on paper. Stable energy then becomes harder to achieve because one of the body's major long-duration fuel sources is not being claimed efficiently. Pancreatic lipase and triglyceride breakdown therefore sit at the center of a larger nutritional truth. A food can be dense in fat and still feed the body poorly if the chemistry of digestion never reaches the point where those lipids are actually liberated.

Micelles, Absorption, and Chylomicrons

Once pancreatic lipase has broken triglycerides into free fatty acids and monoglycerides, the body is still not finished with the problem of fat. The chemistry has changed, but the transport problem remains. These lipid fragments are still hydrophobic. They do not move comfortably through the watery environment of the intestinal lumen on their own, and they cannot simply drift across the absorptive surface in useful quantity without help. This is where micelles matter. Bile acids gather around the products of fat digestion and organize them into tiny transport assemblies with a water-facing exterior and a lipid-carrying interior. In practical terms, micelles are the body's way of ferrying fat through a medium that resists it. They do not digest the fat. They make the digested fat deliverable.

That delivery step is critical because the absorptive surface of the small intestine is not floating out in the middle of the meal. The brush border, the dense microvillus surface of the enterocyte, sits behind a thin unstirred water layer that lipid fragments must cross before they can enter the cell. Micelles solve that last approach. They carry fatty acids, monoglycerides, cholesterol, and fat-soluble vitamins through the aqueous phase and bring them into close contact with the intestinal membrane. At the surface, the lipid cargo leaves the micelle and enters the enterocyte. The bile acids themselves are not absorbed in that moment with the rest of the lipid cargo. They stay in the intestinal lumen and can participate again downstream until they are reclaimed later through enterohepatic recycling. So micelles are temporary carriers, not the final transport form inside the body.

Absorption into the enterocyte changes the problem again. The goal now is no longer to move hydrophobic molecules through intestinal fluid. The goal is to package them for circulation. Inside the absorptive cell, fatty acids and monoglycerides are reassembled into triglycerides. Cholesterol is esterified in part. These lipids are then combined with phospholipids and specialized apolipoproteins to form chylomicrons, large lipoprotein particles built specifically to transport dietary fat after absorption. This is a major shift. In the lumen, bile acids had to keep fat suspended in microscopic mobile form. Inside the cell, the body rebuilds the fat into a denser transport package suitable for internal distribution. Digestion and transport are working in sequence. First disperse. Then hydrolyze. Then ferry. Then rebuild.

Chylomicrons matter because dietary fat cannot enter portal blood the way amino acids and glucose do. They are too large and too lipid-rich for that route. Instead they are secreted from the enterocyte into lacteals, the lymphatic vessels that run through the villi of the small intestine. From there they move through the lymphatic system and only later enter the bloodstream near the heart. This detour explains several important features of fat physiology. It helps explain why dietary fat enters the circulation more gradually than rapidly absorbed carbohydrate. It helps explain why post-meal energy from fat tends to be slower and steadier rather than abrupt. It also shows that fat digestion is not just about cleavage. It is about choreography. The body has to change the form of the nutrient multiple times before that nutrient becomes usable internal fuel and structural material.

This sequence also reveals why breakdown at any step can lower the real value of a fatty meal. If bile flow is poor, micelle formation weakens. If pancreatic lipase activity is impaired, there are fewer lipid fragments to carry. If enterocyte function is compromised, reassembly and packaging into chylomicrons falter. The meal can still contain abundant fat on paper while delivering much less into actual circulation. That is why micelles, absorption, and chylomicrons belong in the same sentence. Together they describe the point where dietary fat stops being food in the lumen and becomes a transportable internal nutrient stream.

Why Fats Enter the Body Differently Than Sugars and Amino Acids

Fats enter the body differently because they do not dissolve into the body's water-based transport system the way sugars and amino acids do. Glucose and amino acids are water-soluble enough to move from the intestinal lumen into enterocytes and then directly into portal blood, the venous system that carries absorbed nutrients straight to the liver. Their route is relatively direct. Digest them, transport them across the intestinal lining, release them into blood, send them to the liver. Fat cannot do that cleanly because its chemistry is different. Fatty acids and the triglycerides they come from are hydrophobic. They resist the aqueous environment of the gut and the bloodstream. The body therefore has to handle them through a separate logistical system built around bile, micelles, intracellular repackaging, and lymphatic transport. That difference is not incidental. It changes the timing of absorption, the speed of nutrient entry into circulation, and the entire post-meal metabolic pattern.

Sugars follow the fastest route. Starches are broken down into simple sugars, sugars cross the intestinal lining through dedicated transporters, and glucose enters portal blood quickly enough that the liver and pancreas have to respond almost immediately. Insulin rises. Glucose is partitioned into current use, glycogen storage, or later fat production depending on the larger metabolic state. Amino acids move differently from glucose, but they still take the same general vascular route. Protein is digested into amino acids and small peptides, these cross the intestinal membrane, and then they enter portal circulation for first-pass handling by the liver. The liver sorts them, uses some, converts some, and releases the rest into wider circulation. Both sugars and amino acids therefore enter the body through a blood-first route that exposes the liver early and directly to what was absorbed.

Fat has to take the long way in because it cannot remain in that simple dissolved state. After bile emulsifies dietary fat and pancreatic lipase hydrolyzes triglycerides into fatty acids and monoglycerides, those lipid fragments are carried through the watery intestinal contents inside micelles. Once they enter the enterocyte, they are not released directly into blood in that form. They are rebuilt into triglycerides and packaged with phospholipids, cholesterol, and apolipoproteins into chylomicrons, large lipoprotein transport particles. Those particles are too large to enter ordinary capillaries, so they are secreted into lacteals, the lymphatic vessels inside the villi of the small intestine. From there they travel through lymph before finally entering the bloodstream near the heart. This means dietary fat bypasses the immediate portal route that sugars and amino acids use. It enters circulation later, in a different package, through a different physical system.

That different route changes physiology. Sugars can create a fast rise in blood glucose because their entry into portal blood is rapid and direct. Amino acids can appear in portal blood quickly as well, though their metabolic meaning is more structural and regulatory than purely energetic. Fat enters more slowly because it must be emulsified, hydrolyzed, repackaged, and carried through lymph before it joins the blood. That slower arrival helps explain why fat-rich meals often produce steadier energy and longer satiety rather than the sharper rise-and-fall pattern more common with refined carbohydrate. The digestive system is not simply absorbing nutrients at different speeds by accident. It is using different transport architectures because the nutrients themselves create different chemical problems and serve different biological roles.

This is also why fat digestion failure can look different from poor carbohydrate or protein handling. If sugar absorption is rapid and excessive, blood glucose and insulin show the strain quickly. If protein digestion is poor, structural underfeeding and upper digestive discomfort may become visible. If fat handling is weak, the problem often appears as poor bile-dependent digestion, greasy stools, heaviness after meals, weak absorption of fat-soluble vitamins, and loss of access to a major stable fuel source. The nutrient is present in the meal, but its route into the body is more complex and therefore easier to disrupt at several stages. Fats enter differently because they have to. Their chemistry forces the body to treat them through a separate absorption and transport system, and that system shapes everything from satiety to energy stability to vitamin delivery.

Why Fat Tends to Create Slower, Steadier Energy Delivery

Fat tends to create slower, steadier energy delivery because the body cannot move it from plate to bloodstream with the speed it uses for refined carbohydrate. Fat has to pass through more gates. It must leave the stomach more slowly, because fat-rich meals delay gastric emptying. It must then be emulsified by bile, hydrolyzed by pancreatic lipase, carried in micelles through the aqueous environment of the small intestine, absorbed into enterocytes, reassembled into triglycerides, packaged into chylomicrons, and sent through the lymphatic system before joining the bloodstream. That sequence takes time. The body is not being flooded with a fast soluble fuel. It is receiving lipid energy through a staged delivery system that stretches the meal out physiologically. The chemistry itself forces a slower pace.

That slower pace changes the hormonal picture. Refined carbohydrate can be broken into glucose quickly and moved directly into portal blood, which means the pancreas often has to answer with a relatively rapid insulin response. Fat does not usually create that same abrupt glucose-insulin event because it is not entering as blood sugar. It is entering as lipid transport. The body still has to decide what to oxidize, what to store, and what tissues should receive incoming fuel, but the signal is broader and less abrupt. This is one reason fat-rich meals often feel more stable once digestion is functioning well. Energy arrives over a longer window, and the organism is not forced into the same rapid containment pattern required by fast carbohydrate exposure.

Fat also tends to slow the meal mechanically and hormonally. In the gut, it stimulates cholecystokinin and related satiety signals, increases the need for bile release, and prolongs digestive contact. That does two things at once. It lengthens nutrient delivery and lengthens satiety. The person is not only receiving fuel more gradually. He is also less likely to feel the rapid drop in satisfaction that often follows meals built around quickly absorbed carbohydrate with weak structural value. Protein often strengthens this effect further when it is present alongside fat, because the meal then provides both structural material and slower fuel.

This does not mean all fat-containing foods are automatically stabilizing. A hyper-palatable processed food built from refined starch, sugar, and industrial fat can still produce a chaotic result because the fast carbohydrate signal and the slower fat signal are colliding inside the same meal. But when fat is delivered in a more coherent meal, especially alongside substantial protein, the body usually experiences it as a longer-burning substrate. The stomach slows down. The intestine works through a bile-dependent sequence. Lymphatic transport stretches delivery. Satiety hormones build. The result is not magic. It is timing. Fat tends to create steadier energy because the body is structurally forced to handle it in a slower, more controlled way.

Why This Matters in a Facultative Carnivore Dietary Pattern

This matters in a facultative carnivore dietary pattern because fat is no longer a decorative macronutrient sitting beside the real food. It becomes one of the central inputs the digestive system is expected to handle well and one of the main fuels the body is expected to rely on between meals. If bile flow is weak, if gallbladder release is poorly timed, if pancreatic lipase activity is inadequate, or if intestinal absorption is compromised, the pattern will feel heavier and less effective than it should. The person may conclude that higher-fat eating does not suit him, when the deeper issue is often that the digestive architecture responsible for lipid handling is underperforming. A facultative carnivore framework depends on animal foods as the structural base, and those foods usually bring significant fat with them. That means the body has to do more than tolerate fat in theory. It has to emulsify it, hydrolyze it, absorb it, and turn it into stable fuel and useful tissue material with high enough efficiency that the meal actually delivers what the pattern is built around.

This is also where the difference between carbohydrate-centered eating and fat-centered eating becomes physiologically visible. In a pattern built around frequent starch and sugar, the body is trained to expect fast glucose entry, repeated insulin handling, and shorter intervals between fuel deliveries. In a facultative carnivore pattern, the rhythm shifts. Meals built around protein and fat are slower. Gastric emptying is slower. Bile release becomes more important. Lymphatic transport becomes more relevant. Satiety is expected to last longer because the meal is delivering dense structural material and slower-moving fuel rather than primarily rapid glucose. That change is not cosmetic. It changes what the body asks of digestion and what the person experiences as normal. Stable energy, lower urgency around eating, and reduced dependence on frequent carbohydrate intake all depend on fat digestion working cleanly enough to make those outcomes real.

It also matters because animal fat is not only fuel in this framework. It is part of the nutritional architecture. Fat carries fat-soluble vitamins, supports bile-responsive digestion, contributes to membrane composition, provides cholesterol and fatty acids for hormone synthesis, and helps create the satiety pattern that makes a protein-and-fat-centered diet sustainable without constant management. If fat digestion is poor, the person loses access to more than calories. He loses part of the system's stability. The meal may still be rich, but less of its value crosses into the body. Vitamins A, D, E, and K are absorbed less efficiently. Satiety may weaken. Energy may feel heavy rather than steady because the digestive burden rose while the nutrient yield fell. In that state, a facultative carnivore pattern can be judged unfairly because the digestive failure is being mistaken for a dietary failure.

This is why fat digestion has to be taken seriously in this context. A facultative carnivore pattern is not simply lower in carbohydrate. It is more dependent on the body's ability to turn animal fat into usable biology. When that ability is intact, the pattern often feels calmer, steadier, and more self-regulating because the meals align better with the body's structural and energetic needs. When that ability is weak, the same meals can feel burdensome. The difference is not ideological. It is digestive. The pattern only works as intended when the liver, gallbladder, pancreas, small intestine, and lymphatic transport system are doing their share of the work.

Chapter 16

Fat Beyond Calories

Fat is not merely something the body burns or stores. A large share of what the body does with fat is architectural. Every cell is bounded by a membrane, and that membrane is built largely from lipids arranged into a bilayer, two facing sheets whose water-loving heads point outward and whose fat-loving tails point inward. This structure is not decorative wrapping. It is the living boundary that allows the cell to remain a cell at all. Without it, there is no controlled interior, no maintained gradients, no signaling interface, no transport gate, no meaningful separation between the chemistry inside the cell and the chemistry outside it. The membrane holds the cell together physically, but it also governs what enters, what leaves, what binds, what gets recognized, and how the cell responds to the world around it. That means dietary fat is never only about calories. Part of it becomes the material out of which these boundaries are built and rebuilt.

The main membrane lipids are phospholipids, molecules with a phosphate-containing head that interacts with water and fatty acid tails that form the hydrophobic interior of the bilayer. Cholesterol sits among them, adding stability and helping control membrane fluidity, the degree to which the membrane remains flexible without becoming leaky or disordered. This balance matters because membranes are not inert walls. Receptors for hormones, neurotransmitters, and immune signals are embedded in them. Ion channels that move sodium, potassium, calcium, and chloride across the membrane depend on the surrounding lipid environment. Transport proteins that carry glucose, amino acids, and other molecules through the membrane are also working inside this structure. If the membrane is poorly built, the cell does not simply become weaker in some vague way. Its signaling changes. Its transport changes. Its electrical behavior changes. Its physical resilience changes.

This is why the type of fat entering the diet matters beyond simple energy accounting. Fatty acids absorbed from food can be incorporated into membrane phospholipids, which means repeated dietary exposure shapes the material properties of the membrane over time. Saturated fats create straighter, more tightly packed tails. Monounsaturated fats create a different structural effect because their single double bond introduces a bend. Polyunsaturated fats create even more bends and greater fluidity, but they are also more chemically reactive because those double bonds are easier targets for oxidation. The body uses a mixture because membranes have to be both stable and dynamic. Too rigid and transport and signaling become impaired. Too unstable and the membrane becomes more vulnerable to oxidative damage and disordered function. Food therefore contributes directly to the physical behavior of cell boundaries. The membrane is not sealed off from diet. It is partly built from it.

This becomes especially important in tissues that depend heavily on precise signaling and high membrane turnover. Nerve tissue relies on lipid-rich structures for insulation, conduction, and receptor behavior. Immune cells need membranes capable of rapid signaling and remodeling. Liver cells, intestinal cells, muscle cells, and endocrine tissues all depend on membranes that can hold gradients, host transport proteins, and respond appropriately to changing metabolic conditions. A diet that repeatedly supplies usable fats in biologically coherent forms supports that work. A diet that reduces fat to a feared calorie source misses the point completely. The body is not just asking whether it has enough fuel. It is asking whether it has the right material to maintain the boundaries through which almost all cellular life is organized.

So when fat is discussed only as stored energy or dietary risk, one of its most basic roles disappears. Fat in cell membranes is not an optional side story. It is part of how the body maintains order. The membrane decides what the cell can keep, what it can reject, what signals it can hear, and how well it can function under stress. Dietary fat reaches that level. It does not merely pass through metabolism as burnable substrate. Some of it becomes structure, and that structure is where much of physiology actually happens.

Fat in Steroid Hormone Production

Fat matters in steroid hormone production because steroid hormones are built from cholesterol, and cholesterol is a lipid molecule, not a carbohydrate, not an amino acid, and not an abstract wellness concept. Testosterone, estrogen, progesterone, cortisol, aldosterone, all of them belong to this steroid family. They do not appear out of thin air because the endocrine system is in a good mood. They are synthesized through a chain of enzymatic conversions that begins with cholesterol and proceeds through tightly regulated steps inside steroid-producing tissues such as the adrenal glands, ovaries, testes, and, in a different but related way, other tissues that participate in steroid metabolism. That means fat is relevant to hormone production at the level of raw substrate. A body chronically underfed in usable lipid material is not merely eating less fat. It is narrowing part of the chemical foundation from which one of its most important hormone classes is made.

The story starts in the membrane. Cholesterol is embedded in cell membranes throughout the body, where it helps regulate fluidity and structural stability, but it is also the precursor that steroidogenic tissues draw on when hormone synthesis is required. Inside those cells, cholesterol is transported into mitochondria, where the first committed step in steroid hormone synthesis begins. There, enzymes convert cholesterol into pregnenolone, the parent steroid from which many other steroid hormones are derived. From pregnenolone, the body branches into multiple pathways depending on tissue type, enzyme expression, and physiological need. One branch leads toward progesterone. Others move toward cortisol, aldosterone, testosterone, and estrogens. This is not casual chemistry. It is a controlled series of transformations that depends on adequate substrate, intact enzyme systems, and a regulatory environment that tells the tissue what kind of hormone output is needed.

This is why dietary fat cannot be reduced honestly to "just energy" when hormone biology is being discussed. The body can synthesize cholesterol internally, yes, but that does not make dietary fat irrelevant. The organism still depends on intact lipid metabolism, adequate fatty acid supply, and membrane health to support the tissues that produce and respond to steroid hormones. Cholesterol synthesis itself depends on broader metabolic status. The membranes that house receptors, transporters, and signaling systems depend on lipid material. Steroid hormones are lipid-derived molecules moving through and acting on a lipid-based cellular architecture. A low-fat framework that ignores this can easily become physiologically thin. The person may still be alive, may still have measurable hormones, may still function at a basic level, but that is not the same as saying the endocrine system is being supported well.

Fatty acids matter here too, even when they are not converted directly into the steroid backbone itself. The endocrine system does not operate in isolation from the rest of metabolism. Membrane composition affects receptor behavior and signal transduction. Inflammatory state affects steroid signaling and tissue sensitivity. Energy sufficiency affects the body's willingness to invest in reproductive function versus stress adaptation. Adipose tissue, liver function, insulin signaling, thyroid status, and nutrient sufficiency all feed back into the steroid system. So when dietary fat is too low, too unstable, or repeatedly displaced by processed carbohydrate, the cost can appear indirectly as well. The body may alter reproductive output, stress response, or downstream hormone balance not because a single dietary fat molecule was missing, but because the larger lipid environment no longer supports calm and coherent endocrine function.

This becomes most obvious when people talk about hormones as though they could be fixed by targeting one blood marker without addressing the material economy underneath it. Steroid hormones are not floating abstractions. They are built from cholesterol, regulated by enzymes, transported through blood, received at membranes, and metabolized by the liver and other tissues. All of that sits inside a body whose cellular architecture is itself lipid-dependent. So when fat in the diet is dismissed, feared, or chronically stripped away, the body is not just losing one fuel source. It is losing part of the substrate base and structural environment required for normal steroid hormone production and signaling. Fat in this context is not indulgence. It is part of the chemistry of endocrine life.

Fat in Nervous System Structure

The nervous system is not built like a dry electrical wire. It is built as living lipid architecture. Neurons, their membranes, their insulating layers, their synaptic interfaces, and much of the machinery that allows signals to move from one cell to another depend heavily on fat. This begins with the membrane itself. Every neuron is bounded by a phospholipid bilayer, a lipid membrane that holds the cell together, maintains ion gradients, anchors receptors and channels, and determines how electrical and chemical signals can be received and transmitted. Sodium, potassium, calcium, and chloride do not move across a neuron because the cell is vaguely alive. They move through proteins embedded in a membrane whose physical properties matter. That membrane must be fluid enough to function, stable enough to hold gradients, and structurally coherent enough to keep signaling precise. Fat is part of what gives it those properties.

The dependence becomes even more obvious in myelin, the lipid-rich insulating sheath wrapped around many nerve fibers. Myelin allows action potentials, the rapid electrical signals that travel along nerves, to move faster and more efficiently by reducing current loss and forcing the signal to jump between nodes of Ranvier rather than leaking continuously along the axon. This is not a minor improvement. It is one of the reasons the nervous system can coordinate movement, reflexes, sensory processing, and thought at the speed it does. Myelin is built largely from lipid material, along with specialized proteins, and maintaining it requires a body that can digest, absorb, transport, and deploy fats effectively. A nervous system stripped of adequate lipid support is not just low on energy. It is underbuilt at the level of insulation and signal conduction.

The brain itself makes the point even harder to ignore. It is rich in lipids because its function depends on them. Neuronal membranes have to host receptors for neurotransmitters, transporters for nutrient and ion handling, and signaling complexes that respond to changing metabolic conditions in milliseconds. Synapses, the junctions where one neuron communicates with another, are membrane-dense environments where vesicles fuse, neurotransmitters are released, receptors are activated, and signaling cascades are initiated. All of that depends on membrane composition. If the membrane environment is poorly maintained, signaling changes. Receptor behavior changes. Transport changes. The speed and clarity of communication can change. Fat in this context is not background fuel sitting off to the side while glucose runs the show. It is part of the physical substrate through which nervous function becomes possible.

Cholesterol matters here as well. It is not only a blood marker or a steroid precursor. It is a structural lipid that helps stabilize membranes and regulate their fluidity, and the nervous system relies on that stability. Cholesterol is abundant in myelin and in neuronal membranes because those structures need a precise balance between flexibility and order. Too rigid and function suffers. Too unstable and the membrane becomes disordered and vulnerable. The body synthesizes cholesterol internally, but that does not make dietary fat irrelevant. Nervous tissue still depends on intact lipid metabolism, adequate essential fatty acid supply, and a broader nutritional environment that supports membrane maintenance and repair.

This is why reducing fat to "just calories" becomes especially misleading when nervous system biology is considered. A person can consume enough energy and still fail to support the lipid architecture that nerves depend on if food quality is poor and structural fats are displaced by low-value processed inputs. The nervous system does not merely need enough fuel to keep firing. It needs membranes that can hold gradients, myelin that can insulate axons, and lipid-rich structural integrity that keeps signaling sharp and coordinated. Fat in nervous system structure is therefore not a luxury. It is part of the material basis of electrical life.

Fat as a Stable Long-Duration Fuel

Fat functions as a stable long-duration fuel because the body does not have to move it through metabolism with the speed and volatility required for rapid glucose handling. Carbohydrate, especially in refined form, often enters circulation quickly, raises blood glucose quickly, and forces the pancreas to answer with insulin quickly. That produces a fast fuel event. Fat behaves differently from the start. It leaves the stomach more slowly, depends on bile for emulsification, requires pancreatic lipase for hydrolysis, enters the body through micelle-mediated absorption, is repackaged into chylomicrons, and travels first through lymphatic circulation before joining the bloodstream. The entire sequence stretches delivery out in time. This is not an accident or a nutritional slogan. It is built into the chemistry and transport route of fat itself. The body is receiving fuel more gradually, and that gradual delivery changes what energy feels like inside the organism.

Once fatty acids are available to tissues, they can be oxidized through beta-oxidation, the mitochondrial process that breaks fatty acid chains into acetyl-CoA units that feed into the citric acid cycle and oxidative phosphorylation. This matters because fat is not merely slower to arrive. It is also dense in stored chemical energy and well suited to sustained ATP production when oxygen is available and metabolic conditions permit. A fatty acid does not create the same abrupt endocrine picture as a large glucose pulse. It does not have to be contained as blood sugar. It can be mobilized, transported, taken up by tissues, and oxidized in a pattern that better supports duration than urgency. That is why a body relying more heavily on fat for fuel often feels steadier between meals. The system is drawing from a substrate that is abundant, energy-dense, and less dependent on repeated feeding intervals to keep supply moving.

This stability shows up partly through the absence of sharp oscillation. Glucose-based metabolism is not inherently pathological, but it is easier to destabilize because blood glucose has to be held within a relatively narrow range. A meal that raises it quickly creates a larger insulin event, and when that fuel is used or stored, the person may feel the drop more distinctly if the meal was weak in protein and fat. Fat does not operate under that same narrow blood-level management problem because it is not circulating as blood sugar. It arrives through a slower route, enters tissues differently, and can be drawn on over longer periods. Combined with adequate protein, this often produces the practical effects people describe as stable energy, fewer crashes, and less urgency around the next meal. The body is not living off a short-burning substrate that needs frequent replenishment. It is running on a fuel that was built for storage and sustained use.

Adipose tissue makes the same point at larger scale. Body fat exists as the major long-term energy reserve because fat stores large amounts of usable energy without the water burden required by glycogen storage. That is one reason humans can carry enough stored fat energy to survive long periods without food while glycogen reserves are comparatively limited. The body would not be designed this way if fat were only a secondary or fragile fuel. The storage architecture itself tells you the priority. Fat is how the organism carries long-range energy security. Dietary fat aligns with that biology because it supplies the same class of substrate the body already relies on for stored fuel.

This is why fat becomes especially important in a dietary pattern built around satiety and metabolic steadiness rather than constant glucose replenishment. It does not merely add calories to the plate. It changes the timing and texture of energy access. It slows the meal, supports bile-driven digestion, extends nutrient delivery, reduces dependence on repeated fast-fuel exposure, and gives the body a substrate it is structurally equipped to burn over longer intervals. Fat as a stable long-duration fuel is therefore not a theory layered onto the body from outside. It is visible in the chemistry of digestion, the route of absorption, the structure of adipose storage, and the mitochondrial pathways that turn fatty acids into sustained energy.

Why Low-Fat Frameworks Misunderstood Basic Physiology

Low-fat frameworks misunderstood basic physiology because they treated fat as a passive danger instead of asking what fat actually does inside the body. They saw energy density, saw circulating lipids, saw stored body fat, and then collapsed all three into a single fear. The conclusion became simple enough for public health messaging. Eat less fat, especially saturated fat, and health will improve. But the body does not experience dietary fat as a moral category or a symbolic risk factor. It experiences fat as membrane material, hormone substrate, bile-dependent digestive input, long-duration fuel, and the carrier required for absorption of fat-soluble vitamins. Once that is understood, the low-fat frame starts looking thin. It did not merely recommend less of one nutrient. It downgraded one of the main structural and regulatory materials the organism uses to keep itself built and stable.

The first mistake was treating dietary fat mainly as stored body fat in waiting. That confuses nutrient class with metabolic fate. Yes, fat can be stored. So can excess carbohydrate after it moves through insulin signaling and hepatic handling. But what matters physiologically is not whether a nutrient can become stored energy. It is what else that nutrient is doing while it is in the system. Dietary fat slows gastric emptying, supports satiety, enters membranes, provides essential fatty acids, contributes to steroid hormone biology, and enables the intestinal absorption of vitamins A, D, E, and K. A low-fat meal can reduce one visible input while increasing another burden. Hunger often rises. Glucose handling becomes more dominant. Refined carbohydrate is often used to replace what fat once supplied in density and palatability. The eater may consume fewer grams of fat while producing weaker satiety and more unstable energy. The framework congratulates itself because one macronutrient fell. The body still has to manage the consequences of what replaced it.

The second mistake was ignoring digestive architecture. Human physiology is not built as if fat were an accidental indulgence. The liver makes bile continuously. The gallbladder stores and concentrates it. The intestine releases cholecystokinin in response to fat. Pancreatic lipase and colipase exist specifically to break triglycerides down. Enterocytes rebuild absorbed lipid fragments into chylomicrons for lymphatic transport. A body does not invest this much coordinated anatomy and chemistry into a nutrient that is metabolically trivial. The existence of a bile system alone should have warned against simplistic low-fat thinking. Fat digestion is not a side pathway. It is a major standing commitment of human physiology. Low-fat frameworks treated that entire architecture as though it were optional background rather than evidence of biological design.

The third mistake was flattening lipid biology into a blood-marker argument. Circulating lipoproteins matter. Cardiovascular risk matters. But those observations do not erase the broader truth that fats differ, foods differ, and the body uses lipid material at every scale from the cell membrane upward. Cholesterol is part of membrane stability and steroid hormone production. Phospholipids form the bilayer of every cell. Myelin in the nervous system is lipid rich. Fatty acids participate in inflammatory signaling and energy production. A low-fat framework that speaks only in the language of risk reduction can miss the more basic issue of what the organism is made from and how it remains intact. It is possible to narrow one laboratory variable while under-supporting the structural biology that makes cellular life function well.

The fourth mistake was misunderstanding appetite. Fat is not only dense in energy. It is part of why meals can feel complete. It extends digestion, slows delivery, and works with protein to create longer satiety. When fat is stripped out and replaced with starches, sugars, and low-structure processed foods, the body often receives faster fuel with weaker completion. Hunger returns sooner. Eating becomes more frequent. Blood glucose becomes a more dominant regulator of mood and energy. The person is then told to show more discipline. But a meal pattern that weakens satiety and speeds fuel turnover is already working against the eater. Low-fat frameworks often blamed appetite dysregulation on personal weakness when the physiology of the meal itself was part of the problem.

The deeper issue is that low-fat thinking reduced nutrition to subtraction when the body needed a materials-based accounting. It asked how much fat could be removed without first asking what fat was doing there. It treated energy density as the main truth and structural function as secondary. That is backward. The body is not maintained by avoiding dense nutrients. It is maintained by receiving the right ones in usable form. Fat can certainly be mishandled in a disordered diet, especially when it appears inside ultra-processed food alongside refined carbohydrate and weak protein. But that is not an argument against fat as such. It is an argument against judging nutrients outside the total physiological event. Low-fat frameworks missed that distinction. They saw fat as a quantity to fear rather than a biological material to understand.

Part V

Nutrient Density, Organs, and Biological Yield

Chapter 17

Energy Density vs Biological Value

Calories are a poor nutritional measure because they describe potential heat, not usable nourishment. A calorie tells you how much energy a food can release under combustion conditions. It does not tell you what digestion had to do to that food, what compounds were actually liberated from the matrix, what remained bound in the gut lumen, what crossed the intestinal membrane, what reached the liver intact, what tissues could use directly, and what the body had to clear afterward. That difference is not academic. It is the difference between paper energy and biological yield. A food can be energy-dense and still nourish poorly if the energy arrives with weak protein, poor micronutrient value, low satiety, unstable glucose handling, or a larger digestive and excretory burden than the label suggests. The body does not live on theoretical heat. It lives on what it can extract, absorb, retain, and use.

This is easiest to see when two foods carry similar energy but create completely different physiological events. A processed snack built from refined flour, sugar, and industrial oil may deliver substantial calories with almost no meaningful structural return. It can digest quickly, raise blood glucose quickly, provoke insulin quickly, and still leave the organism underfed where it matters. Complete amino acids are scarce. Fat-soluble nutrients are weak. Mineral density is poor or synthetic. Satiety is short-lived because the meal supplied fast fuel more effectively than it supplied durable nourishment. By contrast, a meal built from meat, eggs, dairy, or other nutrient-dense animal foods may carry equal or greater calories while delivering complete protein, usable fats, bioavailable minerals, and longer satiety. The calorie number does not capture that difference because the calorie number is blind to what the body is actually receiving.

Calories also ignore digestive cost. The body does not extract nutrition for free. It spends acid, enzymes, bile, membrane transport, liver handling, and renal clearance on every meal. A food that requires more work while yielding less usable nutrition is biologically inferior even if its calorie count looks efficient. Plant foods can illustrate this sharply. A food may test rich in minerals or protein while packaging those nutrients inside fiber, phytate, lectins, oxalate, or other compounds that reduce access. The label preserves the nutrient claim. The intestine delivers much less. The same problem appears in processed food from the opposite direction. The meal may be easy to absorb as energy, but that ease often reflects refinement, not nourishment. Quick absorption is not the same as good feeding. Sometimes it means the food has been stripped down to a form that burdens glucose control while underdelivering structure.

The deeper failure of calorie thinking is that it reduces the body to an energy sink instead of a living construction project. Human physiology depends on proteins for enzymes, connective tissue, immune defense, and repair. It depends on fats for membranes, steroid hormone production, nervous system structure, and stable fuel. It depends on vitamins and minerals for enzyme function, redox control, oxygen transport, and cellular signaling. None of that disappears because a food contains measurable energy. A person can consume plenty of calories and still remain biologically undernourished if the incoming food keeps solving the energy problem while failing the structural one. That is one of the defining features of the modern processed diet. The body is fed and unfinished at the same time.

So calories can tell you something narrow. They can estimate how much fuel a food might provide. They cannot tell you whether the food is worth eating as a biological input. For that you need a harder standard. What did digestion release. What reached the blood. What supported tissue. What stabilized appetite. What burdened clearance. What was the body left with after the full event was over. That is nutritional value. The calorie count is only one small shadow cast by it.

The Difference Between Energy and Usable Structure

Energy and usable structure are not the same biological thing, even when they arrive in the same meal. Energy is what the body can burn. Usable structure is what the body can build with. A food may provide one without providing much of the other. Sugar can deliver rapid energy with almost no structural value. Refined starch can do the same on a slightly longer timeline. Industrial fat can add dense calories to a product while contributing little to the broader nutritional architecture if the rest of the food is weak. The body can run on that input for a while, but running is not the same as being maintained. Cells do not rebuild membranes from calories in the abstract. Enzymes are not synthesized from heat units. Connective tissue is not repaired by arithmetic. The organism needs amino acids for proteins, fatty acids and cholesterol for membranes and steroid hormone synthesis, minerals for electrical gradients and enzyme function, and vitamins as cofactors that allow the machinery to run. When food delivers energy without enough of that structural material, the body is fueled and underbuilt at the same time.

This is why the modern diet can produce the strange condition of abundance without real sufficiency. A person can eat enough or even too much in caloric terms and still fail to supply the tissues properly. Hunger may persist because the body solved the immediate fuel problem but not the construction problem. Recovery may weaken because enough substrate never arrived to rebuild what daily life keeps wearing down. Hair, skin, connective tissue, lean mass, immune resilience, and metabolic stability all begin to reflect the same deficit from different angles. The body is not asking only whether energy came in. It is asking what kind of material crossed the intestinal membrane, what can be retained, and what can be turned into living structure once the meal is over. That is the distinction calorie language usually hides. A food can be good at keeping the organism running for the next few hours and bad at helping the organism remain well built over the next few years.

Animal foods often clarify this difference because they tend to deliver both sides of the equation at once. Protein comes with complete amino acid patterns the body can use directly for tissue maintenance. Fat arrives as usable lipid material for membranes, signaling, and slower fuel delivery. Minerals and fat-soluble vitamins often come in forms digestion can access with relatively high yield. Many processed foods do the opposite. They separate energy from architecture. They deliver quickly metabolizable fuel through refined carbohydrate and extracted fat while leaving protein thin, micronutrients weak, and satiety incomplete. So the meal may feel substantial for a moment while contributing little to the body's ongoing structural work. The eater gets calories. The tissues get a poor invoice.

That is why usable structure is the higher standard. Energy matters because the body must produce adenosine triphosphate, ATP, continuously to stay alive. But the machinery that produces ATP is itself built from structure. Mitochondrial enzymes are proteins. Membranes are lipid-rich. Transport systems require minerals and protein scaffolds. Blood carries oxygen through iron-containing hemoglobin. Hormones require substrate and signaling architecture. Nothing in metabolism escapes this rule. The body can burn food today and still weaken if the food does not also help replace what the body is made of. So the real nutritional question is never just how much energy a food contains. It is whether that food also contributes the material the organism needs to remain intact while using that energy.

Why Processed Foods Can Overfeed and Undernourish at the Same Time

Processed foods can overfeed and undernourish at the same time because they are built to deliver energy efficiently while delivering structural value poorly. That is the core design problem. Refined flour, sugar, extracted oils, flavor systems, emulsifiers, and soft textures make it easy for large amounts of fuel to enter the body quickly. The digestive work is often reduced in the wrong places. Starch is stripped of much of its original resistance. Sugar arrives already close to absorbable form. Fats are blended into products that require little chewing and create high energy density with very little physical friction. The mouth receives intensity. The gut receives a fast-moving fuel package. But speed of fuel delivery is not the same as nourishment. A processed food can move a substantial calorie load into circulation while supplying weak protein, poor micronutrient density, weak satiety, and very little of the material the body actually uses to rebuild tissue. The person is overfed in energy and underfed in structure during the same meal.

This becomes clearer when the body's real priorities are placed back into view. The organism does not merely need fuel for the next hour. It needs amino acids for enzymes, muscle maintenance, immune proteins, gut lining turnover, connective tissue repair, and transport proteins. It needs fats for membranes, nervous system structure, steroid hormone production, and fat-soluble vitamin absorption. It needs minerals and vitamins as cofactors for oxidative metabolism, oxygen handling, electrical gradients, and cellular signaling. Most processed foods do not solve these needs well. They solve shelf life, repeat purchase, texture, and reward. A sweetened cereal, flavored snack bar, chips, pastries, frozen desserts, and many packaged convenience foods can all provide substantial energy while contributing little complete protein and only thin or synthetic micronutrient support. Fortification can decorate the label, but fortification does not change the deeper architecture of the meal. The food may still behave primarily as rapidly available fuel with low structural yield.

This is why appetite often remains active after processed food intake. The body received calories, but it may not have received enough complete amino acids, enough useful fats, enough minerals, or enough lasting satiety signals to interpret the meal as biologically complete. Blood glucose may rise quickly. Insulin may rise quickly. Reward in the mouth may be strong. Yet the deeper nutritional request remains partly unresolved. That is why a person can eat a large volume of processed food and still feel strangely unfinished. The meal answered the energy problem first and the structural problem badly or not at all. The brain and gut then keep driving intake because the organism is still searching for what the previous meal failed to supply. This is not mysterious. It is what happens when food is designed to maximize consumption rather than maximize biological completion.

The overfeeding side of the problem is therefore not separate from the undernourishment side. They help create each other. Weak satiety makes repeated intake more likely. Rapid fuel delivery makes blood sugar and appetite less stable. Low protein density means more food volume may be eaten before structural needs are met. Poor micronutrient value means the body keeps receiving energy without enough of the cofactors required to use that energy cleanly. The person is then blamed for overeating, when the food itself was built to create exactly this mismatch between energetic load and nutritional resolution. Processed food overfeeds because it delivers easy calories. It undernourishes because it delivers too little of what the body is actually made from.

Why Nutrient Sufficiency Changes Appetite Behavior

Appetite changes when nutrient sufficiency changes because hunger is not only a request for energy. It is also a response to whether the last meal actually solved the body's material needs. A person can consume substantial calories and still remain biologically unfinished if the meal delivered fast fuel without enough complete protein, useful fat, minerals, or other regulatory nutrients required for repair and stable function. In that state, the appetite system has no reason to quiet down simply because a numerical energy target was reached. The stomach may have been filled for a while. Blood glucose may have risen. Reward may have been generated in the mouth and brain. But the deeper question remains open. Did enough amino acids enter circulation to support protein synthesis. Did enough fat arrive to support membrane maintenance, hormone biology, and sustained satiety. Did the meal provide a micronutrient environment strong enough to support energy metabolism rather than just provoke it. Appetite behaves differently when the answer is yes because the body is no longer being forced to keep searching through repeated intake for materials it failed to get the first time.

Protein is one of the clearest examples because it helps close the structural side of the hunger signal. The body does not keep a large reserve pool of free amino acids, and it depends on repeated intake to maintain muscle, enzymes, immune molecules, connective tissue, gut lining turnover, and repair throughout the organism. When a meal provides enough digestible, complete protein, amino acids rise in the bloodstream in a way that tells the body real building material has arrived. Satiety hormones rise. Gastric emptying remains slower. The meal feels more finished. When protein is weak, diluted, incomplete, or poorly digested, appetite often stays louder because the structural request was not fully answered. The person may interpret that as weak discipline. The physiology is simpler. The body is still waiting for substrate.

Fat changes appetite behavior in a different but equally important way. It slows gastric emptying, increases the release of cholecystokinin and related satiety signals, and extends the timeline of digestion so the body receives a more prolonged post-meal fuel stream rather than a short burst followed by rapid decline. That matters because a meal built around protein and fat tends to supply both structure and slower energy at the same time. The body is not only less empty. It is less metabolically urgent. By contrast, a meal high in refined carbohydrate and low in meaningful structural value may move quickly, raise blood glucose quickly, and leave the eater under-signaled and under-supplied once the rapid fuel has been contained. Hunger then returns sooner, not because the person is irrational, but because the meal resolved the easiest problem first and left the deeper ones open.

Micronutrient sufficiency changes appetite behavior more quietly, but it still matters. Energy production depends on minerals and vitamins acting as cofactors in mitochondrial metabolism, oxygen handling, neurotransmitter synthesis, thyroid signaling, and countless enzymatic reactions. If the diet keeps delivering calories without enough magnesium, zinc, iron, copper, B vitamins, and other regulatory nutrients, the person may remain energetically unstable even while eating enough or too much. The body then keeps pulling toward more food because the incoming energy is not being converted into stable function with enough efficiency. Appetite in that context is not always a direct request for more calories. Often it is the downstream behavior of a body still trying to complete a meal biochemically.

This is why nutrient sufficiency often makes eating feel calmer. When meals consistently deliver enough complete protein, enough useful fat, and enough nutrient density to support real digestion, absorption, and tissue use, appetite stops having to compensate so aggressively. The person may go longer between meals without strain. Cravings may soften. The constant mental noise around food may drop because the body is receiving clearer satiety signals and stronger material support. This does not mean appetite becomes perfect or that reward, habit, emotion, and food engineering cease to matter. It means the biological pressure underneath them is lower. A body that has actually been fed behaves differently from a body that has merely been given calories.

Chapter 18

Fat-Soluble Vitamins and the Lipid Matrix

Vitamins A, D, E, and K are called fat-soluble because the body cannot handle them the way it handles water-soluble nutrients such as vitamin C or many of the B vitamins. They do not move comfortably through the watery environment of the intestine or bloodstream on their own. Their absorption depends on the same digestive machinery used for dietary fat. Bile acids have to emulsify the meal. Lipases and other digestive events have to create the right intestinal conditions. Micelles have to form so these vitamins can be carried through the aqueous contents of the small intestine to the absorptive surface. Enterocytes, the absorptive cells lining the intestine, then take them in and package them into lipid transport particles for movement through the lymphatic system. That means these vitamins are not simply present in a food and then automatically available to the body. Their delivery is tied to fat digestion from the beginning. If bile flow is poor, if fat absorption is weak, or if the meal is structurally wrong for lipid handling, the body may underabsorb them even when intake on paper looks respectable.

This matters because these vitamins do not function like optional decorative extras riding alongside the major nutrients. Vitamin A supports epithelial integrity, vision chemistry, immune regulation, and cellular differentiation, the process by which cells mature into the forms and functions they are meant to carry out. Vitamin D acts more like a hormone than a simple vitamin, influencing calcium handling, immune behavior, and a wide range of gene-level responses. Vitamin E functions as a lipid-phase antioxidant, helping protect polyunsaturated fatty acids and membrane structures from oxidation. Vitamin K is central to blood clotting and to proteins involved in calcium placement, meaning where calcium is directed and retained in the body rather than simply how much calcium is present. These are major regulatory compounds working in membranes, blood, bone, liver, immune tissue, and other systems where lipid handling matters. The body does not need them in huge bulk, but it needs them delivered properly and repeatedly.

The phrase fat-dependent nutrient therefore has two meanings at once. First, these vitamins often arrive in foods that naturally contain fat, especially animal foods such as egg yolks, liver, dairy fat, and certain seafoods. Second, even when they are present, they still depend on dietary fat and intact lipid digestion for absorption. This is why a low-fat meal can distort nutrient delivery in ways that the label never reveals. A person may eat foods containing vitamins A, D, E, and K, or may even swallow a supplement containing them, and still absorb less than expected if the meal does not trigger adequate bile release or if the digestive context is too thin in fat to support normal micelle formation. The nutrient is there. The delivery system is weak. That gap between presence and absorption is one of the reasons simplistic nutrient accounting fails so often in real physiology.

Animal foods tend to matter here because they often provide these vitamins inside a natural lipid matrix rather than as isolated additions sprayed onto processed food. The vitamin is not floating alone. It is arriving with fat, phospholipids, cholesterol, and a broader set of biologically coherent signals that tell the body a lipid-rich meal has arrived and fat digestion should proceed. That does not mean every animal food is equally rich in all four vitamins, or that plant foods contribute nothing at all. It means the body often receives these nutrients most efficiently when they are embedded in foods that already match the requirements of lipid digestion and absorption. By contrast, a fortified low-fat product may preserve the appearance of nutrient adequacy while weakening the very digestive pathway required to absorb what was added.

This is why fat-soluble vitamins cannot be understood honestly outside the lipid matrix. They are not independent passengers. They ride with fat, depend on fat, and are absorbed through the same bile-driven, micelle-mediated sequence that makes dietary lipid usable. A body that fears fat, strips fat away indiscriminately, or handles bile poorly does not simply change its energy pattern. It changes access to an entire class of regulatory nutrients that work at the level of membranes, hormones, oxidation control, coagulation, and tissue maintenance. The vitamin may still be listed. The body may still receive less.

Why Absorption Depends on Bile, Pancreatic Enzymes, and Intact Lipid Handling

Fat-soluble nutrients are not absorbed because they are present in the meal. They are absorbed only if the body can move them through the full lipid-digestion sequence without losing control of the chemistry. That sequence begins with bile. Dietary fat enters the intestine as a water-repelling mass, and vitamins A, D, E, and K are riding inside that lipid environment. If bile acids do not arrive in sufficient quantity, the meal is not properly emulsified. Large fat droplets remain large. Surface area stays low. Pancreatic lipase cannot reach enough of the triglyceride mass to break it down efficiently. The problem begins there. Before the intestine can absorb these vitamins, the meal has to be physically reorganized into microscopic droplets and then into micelles, the tiny transport assemblies that carry lipid digestion products and fat-soluble compounds through the watery contents of the small intestine to the absorptive surface. Without bile, the nutrients may still be in the gut. They are simply stranded there.

Pancreatic enzymes matter because emulsification alone does not finish the job. Bile makes fat accessible. Pancreatic lipase is what cuts triglycerides into free fatty acids and monoglycerides, the smaller lipid units the intestine can actually work with. Colipase helps that lipase stay attached to the fat-water interface so hydrolysis can proceed efficiently. If this enzymatic step is weak, fat remains only partly digested, which means micelle formation weakens and delivery of fat-soluble vitamins to the brush border falls with it. The meal may look rich in lipids and rich in vitamins on paper, but the intestine does not absorb paper. It absorbs what digestion has made transportable. Poor pancreatic contribution lowers that yield.

Intact lipid handling means the whole chain has to remain functional after digestion as well. The products of fat digestion have to be brought to the enterocyte, the absorptive cell lining the small intestine, taken into the cell, and then repackaged into chylomicrons for lymphatic transport. If the enterocyte is inflamed, if bile acid delivery is poor, if pancreatic output is insufficient, or if the body is failing at the later packaging and transport steps, absorption can still falter even when some digestion occurred. This is why fat-soluble vitamin deficiency or poor fat tolerance is not always a problem of low intake. Sometimes the body is eating enough and extracting too little because the lipid-handling machinery is compromised at one or more points in the sequence.

This dependency is what makes low-fat or impaired-fat-digestion states so nutritionally important. Vitamins A, D, E, and K are not absorbed through an independent side door. They depend on the same bile-driven, enzyme-dependent, micelle-mediated pathway used for dietary fat. If bile flow is weak, if pancreatic lipase is underperforming, or if the intestine is not handling lipid transport cleanly, these vitamins fall in value no matter how impressive the label looks. The meal can contain them. The body may still receive much less. That is why absorption depends on bile, pancreatic enzymes, and intact lipid handling. The nutrients do not merely need to be eaten. They need a functioning fat-digestion system to become biologically real.

How Modern Diets Disrupt Delivery of These Nutrients

Modern diets disrupt delivery of fat-soluble vitamins first by breaking the meal away from the digestive conditions those vitamins depend on. Vitamins A, D, E, and K do not move into the body by simple presence. They need fat in the meal, bile release, pancreatic lipase activity, micelle formation, enterocyte uptake, and chylomicron transport. But many modern meals are built in ways that weaken that entire sequence. Some strip natural fat out and then add vitamins back into low-fat products as if the nutrient and the absorption pathway were separate issues. They are not. A fortified skim product, a fat-reduced snack, or a processed meal built around refined starch and low structural fat may preserve the appearance of nutritional adequacy while failing to trigger the same bile response and lipid-handling environment required for efficient absorption. The vitamin is present. The delivery system is underpowered.

The disruption also comes from replacing natural food matrices with industrial ones. In a coherent animal food, fat-soluble vitamins often arrive inside a lipid environment that already fits the body's digestive logic. Egg yolk, liver, dairy fat, certain seafoods, and other animal foods bring the vitamin together with fat, phospholipids, cholesterol, and the chemical context that tells the intestine a real lipid meal has arrived. Many processed foods do the opposite. They isolate components, remove native fat, alter structure, and then patch the product back together with fortification. That may improve the label. It does not guarantee the intestine will see the same biological event. The body is not responding to the nutrient panel. It is responding to what reached the duodenum, what triggered bile release, what formed micelles, and what actually crossed the membrane.

Another problem is that modern diets often damage the organs and processes lipid absorption depends on. A pattern built around frequent refined carbohydrate, sugar-heavy intake, industrial oils, alcohol, and ultra-processed food can burden the liver, disturb bile quality, alter gallbladder rhythm, and create intestinal conditions that make fat handling less efficient. If bile flow is weak, emulsification weakens. If pancreatic contribution is poor, triglyceride breakdown weakens. If the intestinal surface is inflamed or chronically irritated, uptake and transport weaken. The result is not only digestive discomfort after richer meals. The result is that vitamins A, D, E, and K become harder to deliver even when intake appears adequate. A person can be eating foods that contain them, or swallowing supplements that contain them, while the body keeps underreceiving because the machinery of absorption is being disrupted upstream.

Modern eating patterns also create a timing problem. Fat-soluble vitamins are absorbed best when they arrive with a meal substantial enough to activate real fat digestion. But modern eating is often built around grazing, snacking, sweet drinks, protein bars, fortified cereals, low-fat convenience foods, and isolated supplement use detached from proper meal context. That pattern weakens the digestive signal. Instead of one coherent meal that says fat is here, release bile, activate lipid handling, and absorb what came with it, the body gets scattered nutrient exposure with thinner physiological commitment. The vitamins may pass through the gut in a meal too small, too refined, too low in natural fat, or too disordered in composition to deliver them well.

This is why modern diets can look nutritionally advanced and still perform badly at the level of real nutrient delivery. The products are enriched, fortified, labeled, and reformulated, yet the body still needs the same old sequence to make fat-soluble nutrients biologically real. It still needs bile. It still needs pancreatic enzymes. It still needs intact micelle formation. It still needs a healthy absorptive surface. It still needs food that arrives in a form worth digesting. Modern diets often damage that sequence while pretending to replace it with packaging. The result is a nutritional mirage. The vitamin count survives. The body gets less.

Why Natural Fats and Animal Foods Restore Their Biological Context

Natural fats and animal foods restore the biological context of fat-soluble nutrition because they deliver these nutrients inside the same matrix the digestive system was built to handle. Vitamins A, D, E, and K do not function like dry additives that can be sprinkled onto any food and expected to behave the same way. They are lipid-associated compounds. They need fat in the meal, bile release in the intestine, micelle formation in the lumen, and chylomicron transport after absorption. Animal foods often provide that whole sequence in one package. Egg yolk does not give vitamin A in isolation. Liver does not give retinol, copper, and other nutrients in a vacuum. Full-fat dairy does not separate its lipid fraction from the compounds that depend on it. The nutrient arrives with the fat that helps trigger its own digestion and absorption. That is biological context. The food is carrying both the payload and part of the delivery system.

This matters because digestion is not reading the nutrition panel as a list of independent achievements. It is responding to the meal as a physical event. Natural fats entering the duodenum stimulate cholecystokinin, gallbladder contraction, bile release, and the downstream sequence required for lipid handling. Once bile enters, fat is emulsified, lipase gains access, micelles form, and the intestine can begin claiming not only fatty acids and cholesterol but also the fat-soluble vitamins riding with them. In a natural animal food, these events reinforce one another. The meal says fat is here, structural material is here, fat-soluble compounds are here, digest accordingly. A fortified low-fat product says something weaker and less coherent. The vitamin may be present, but the surrounding digestive logic has been thinned out or broken apart.

Animal foods also restore context because they place lipid-soluble nutrients inside tissue rather than inside industrial formulation. The body is not receiving a reconstructed health claim. It is receiving nutrients embedded in a biological substance that once functioned inside another organism. That does not make animal food magical. It makes it integrated. The fats, phospholipids, cholesterol, fat-soluble vitamins, and protein arrive in a form the digestive tract can recognize as a substantial meal rather than a chemically decorated product. This often improves yield because the body is no longer being asked to absorb isolated compounds from a structurally confused food matrix. It is being asked to process real tissue, real fat, real yolk, real milk fat, real organ matter.

The chemistry is still complex, but it is coherent.

This coherence matters beyond absorption alone. Natural fats and animal foods do not simply carry vitamins A, D, E, and K. They often arrive with the broader nutrients that help those compounds make biological sense once absorbed. Retinol in liver arrives inside a food that is also rich in protein and minerals. Egg yolk brings fat-soluble nutrients alongside phospholipids and cholesterol. Dairy fat delivers lipids in a matrix that also contains protein and calcium-containing fractions elsewhere in the food. The body is not just receiving one molecule. It is receiving a network of related materials that participate in membrane biology, hormone production, immune regulation, mineral handling, and tissue maintenance together. This is another part of biological context that modern nutrition keeps flattening. Real foods often deliver systems, not isolated features.

That is why natural fats and animal foods restore something modern diets repeatedly break. They reunite the nutrient with the medium that helps the body absorb it, and they reunite the meal with the digestive signals that make the extraction sequence work properly. Instead of stripped-down products with added claims, the body gets foods that still carry their own physiological logic. The fat tells the gallbladder to release bile. The bile helps absorb the vitamin. The protein supports structure. The lipid matrix supports transport. The organism gets the nutrient in a form that still belongs to a real digestive event. That is what restoration means here. Not nostalgia. Not ideology. A return to foods that still make biological sense when they reach the gut.

Chapter 19

Organ Meats and Whole-Animal Nutrition

Muscle meat and organ meat are not nutritionally interchangeable even though both come from the same animal. Muscle is built primarily for contraction, force production, and movement. Its chemistry reflects that job. It is rich in structural protein, water, and varying amounts of fat depending on the cut and the animal. It provides substantial amino acids, useful minerals, and in many cases a strong base of highly digestible nutrition. But muscle is not where the animal concentrates many of its most metabolically active compounds. Organs are different because organs are working tissues. The liver is processing, storing, converting, and detoxifying. The heart is contracting continuously with dense mitochondrial demand. The kidney is filtering and regulating. These tissues are not just made of protein. They are biochemical centers, and their nutrient density reflects that workload. This is why organ meats can carry far higher concentrations of certain vitamins, minerals, cofactors, and specialized compounds than ordinary muscle meat.

The difference begins with function. Muscle needs amino acids for contractile fibers, some minerals for electrical activity and oxygen handling, and enough energy substrate to perform work. That makes it valuable, especially as a protein source. But organ tissue is metabolically busier and therefore nutritionally denser in a different way. Liver stores vitamin A, concentrates copper, participates in iron handling, and carries a wide range of enzymes and cofactors involved in amino acid metabolism, glucose handling, bile production, and detoxification. Heart muscle is still muscle, but it is a specialized one with continuous oxidative demand and a distinctive nutrient profile. Kidney tissue reflects a filtering and regulatory role. When these tissues are eaten, the body is not only receiving protein. It is receiving the biochemical density of highly active organs.

This is why muscle meat can form a strong nutritional base while still leaving some gaps that organ foods help close. A person living on muscle meat alone can obtain excellent protein, good iron in many cases, zinc, B vitamins, and often a useful fat supply depending on the cut. That already places muscle meat above many plant foods in direct biological yield. But the nutrient distribution across an animal is not flat. Certain vitamins and trace minerals are stored or concentrated more heavily in organs because that is where the animal itself needed them most. Eating only muscle therefore gives the body a large share of structural input without always giving it the full spectrum of concentrated regulatory input that whole-animal eating can provide.

The importance of organ density is easy to misunderstand because modern nutrition often treats foods as if they should all be eaten in similar volume. Organ meats do not work that way. Their density means they are not simply stronger versions of muscle meat to be eaten in the same quantity. They are concentrated tissues. A relatively small amount can contribute substantial vitamin and mineral value because the food is carrying the metabolic intensity of the organ it came from. That is why liver feels categorically different from steak. It is not just another cut. It is a storage and processing organ turned into food. The body receives a different kind of density from it.

So the contrast is not muscle meat bad, organ meat good. That frame would be too shallow. The better contrast is structural density versus regulatory density. Muscle meat is the major protein foundation. It feeds the body's demand for amino acids, supports satiety, and delivers highly usable nutrition with relatively low digestive friction. Organ meats add a different layer. They concentrate nutrients tied to high metabolic activity and storage. Whole-animal nutrition matters because an animal is not made of one uniform tissue, and the nutritional value of eating that animal is not uniform either. Muscle builds the base. Organs widen the range.

Liver and Other Organs as Concentrated Regulatory Nutrition

Liver and other organs matter because they do not merely provide calories or bulk protein. They provide concentrated regulatory nutrition, meaning nutrients tied directly to metabolic control, enzymatic work, oxygen handling, redox balance, detoxification, blood formation, and tissue maintenance. Muscle meat is structurally valuable. It supplies protein, fat, iron, zinc, and a strong amino acid base. But organ tissues are where the animal was actively storing, converting, filtering, synthesizing, and regulating. Their nutrient density reflects those jobs. When the liver is eaten, the body is not just receiving another serving of meat. It is receiving the concentrated biochemical inventory of a tissue that handled vitamin storage, bile production, amino acid metabolism, glycogen regulation, heme turnover, and detoxification chemistry. That concentration is exactly why organ foods feel different nutritionally. They are not more of the same. They are different tissue with different functional density.

Liver makes the case most clearly. It is rich in preformed vitamin A, the retinol form the body can use directly without relying on plant carotene conversion. It carries substantial amounts of vitamin B12, folate, copper, iron, riboflavin, and other cofactors tied to blood production, methylation, oxidative metabolism, and cellular repair. Those are not random nutrients assembled into a convenient package. They are part of what the liver itself needed in order to process amino acids, build plasma proteins, manage nitrogen, support bile chemistry, and carry out its constant sorting work. When the body eats liver, it is consuming a tissue built around metabolic management, and the nutrient profile shows it. This is why liver often corrects thin, low-density eating patterns so sharply. A small amount delivers compounds that do real regulatory work rather than simply expanding the calorie count.

Other organs contribute their own versions of the same logic. Heart is a continuously contracting oxidative organ, and its tissue reflects sustained mitochondrial demand and a high need for energy-handling chemistry. Kidney reflects filtration and biochemical sorting. Spleen, where used traditionally, reflects blood-rich tissue and iron handling. Brain is a distinct case because it is highly lipid-rich and structurally specialized. None of these organs should be treated as interchangeable, and none should be romanticized as magic foods. The point is simpler. Different organs concentrate different aspects of biological function, and eating them widens nutrient coverage in ways muscle alone does not fully reproduce. Whole-animal eating is not valuable because it feels ancestral or complete in a symbolic sense. It is valuable because an animal distributes nutrients unevenly across tissues according to function, and eating only one tissue means accepting that unevenness while leaving some of the richest regulatory fractions unused.

This is especially important in a nutritional culture that keeps separating nutrients from tissues and then wondering why food has become harder to interpret. Modern eating often tries to reconstruct what whole tissues once supplied naturally. Vitamin A is added here. Iron is added there. B12 is taken separately. Folate is discussed in isolation. But in organ foods these compounds arrive already assembled inside a living matrix that digestion can process as food rather than as a list of disconnected interventions. Protein comes with the cofactors that help protein metabolism. Iron comes inside a tissue already built around blood handling. Fat-soluble compounds arrive in a context where lipid digestion can actually deliver them. That coherence does not make organ meats automatically necessary in large amounts, but it does make them biologically distinct. The body is not just receiving nutrients. It is receiving functional tissue.

This is why liver and other organs are best understood as concentrated regulatory nutrition rather than as exotic superfoods. They support the systems that keep metabolism organized. They help fill in nutrient domains tied to blood, energy, detoxification, methylation, and tissue signaling. They do so in small amounts because their density is high. A little liver is not nutritionally equivalent to a little extra lean muscle meat. The organ is carrying a different biochemical job, and the eater inherits that density when it becomes food. Muscle gives the body much of its structural base. Organs deepen the metabolic picture.

Why Nose-to-Tail Eating Changes Micronutrient Coverage

Nose-to-tail eating changes micronutrient coverage because an animal does not distribute nutrients evenly across its body. Different tissues hold different biochemical jobs, and the nutrient map follows that function. Muscle meat is dense in protein and often strong in iron, zinc, and certain B vitamins, but it is not the whole animal's nutritional profile compressed into one uniform tissue. The liver stores and processes. The heart sustains constant oxidative work. Bone and marrow participate in mineral and connective structures. Skin and connective tissues carry collagen-rich architecture. Fat stores lipid-soluble compounds and changes the energy profile of the meal. When a person eats only muscle meat, he is eating the tissue built mainly for movement. When he eats more of the animal, he widens the range of biological functions represented on the plate, and that changes the micronutrient picture immediately.

The clearest example is liver because it concentrates nutrients tied to regulation and storage rather than contraction. Preformed vitamin A, copper, vitamin B12, folate, riboflavin, and other compounds rise sharply there because the liver itself needed them to manage amino acid turnover, bile production, glucose storage, detoxification, heme handling, and plasma protein synthesis. Heart reflects a different physiology. It is still muscle, but it is a highly oxidative one with constant energetic demand and a distinct micronutrient profile. Bone, marrow, skin, and connective tissues expand the intake of collagen-rich proteins and minerals in ways pure lean muscle does not. Fatty tissues alter delivery of fat-soluble vitamins and the overall lipid context of the meal. So nose-to-tail eating does not create a vague sense of completeness by tradition alone. It changes what chemistry actually enters the body because more of the animal's functional geography is being consumed.

This matters because micronutrient deficiency is often a problem of narrow food sourcing, not just low total intake. A person can eat enough calories, enough protein, and enough of one prized food while still repeating the same nutrient pattern day after day. Muscle meat alone gives a strong structural base, but the body's regulatory systems ask for more than structural protein. They ask for retinol, copper, folate, B12, iron, zinc, selenium, riboflavin, vitamin K2 in some animal foods, and a wider distribution of cofactors that support blood production, mitochondrial metabolism, thyroid activity, detoxification, collagen maintenance, and immune signaling. Once more of the animal is eaten, the diet starts covering more of those domains naturally instead of leaning so heavily on fortification, supplementation, or hopeful dietary diversity from lower-yield sources.

Nose-to-tail eating also changes the biological context in which these nutrients arrive. The compounds are not sprinkled onto processed food or swallowed as isolated capsules. They are embedded in real tissue, packaged alongside protein, fat, and other nutrients that often improve the coherence of digestion and absorption. Liver delivers retinol inside an animal matrix already built around storage and metabolism. Marrow and fatty tissues deliver lipids in a context that supports fat-soluble nutrient handling. Connective tissues bring glycine-rich collagen fractions alongside minerals and protein. The body is not receiving a list. It is receiving integrated tissue. That does not guarantee perfection, and it does not mean every organ must be eaten in large amounts, but it does mean the nutritional event becomes broader and more biologically coherent.

This is why nose-to-tail eating changes micronutrient coverage so much more than people expect. It is not just culinary thrift. It is a move away from treating one tissue as though it represented the whole animal nutritionally. The more of the animal's working tissues that are included, the more the diet reflects the animal's full biochemical range. Muscle builds the structural base. Organs widen the regulatory supply. Fat changes the lipid matrix. Connective tissues add a different protein economy. The result is not symbolic completeness. It is a broader nutrient field entering the body in forms digestion can often use with high yield.

Practical Integration of Organs Into a Modern Diet

The practical mistake is to treat organ meats as either mandatory in heroic amounts or too strange to eat at all. Neither frame is useful. Organs are concentrated tissues, which means they should be integrated according to density, not according to the serving size people are used to with steak or ground beef. Liver is the clearest example. It is not just another cut of meat. It is a storage and processing organ rich in preformed vitamin A, copper, vitamin B12, folate, riboflavin, and other regulatory nutrients, so a small amount goes a long way. In practice, this means organs work best as strategic inclusions rather than as the bulk of the diet. Muscle meat still carries most of the daily structural load through complete protein, iron, zinc, and usable fat. Organs widen micronutrient coverage and deepen the regulatory side of the diet. They are additions with force, not filler.

The easiest way to integrate them is to match the organ to the eater's tolerance and to the tissue's nutritional intensity. Liver is usually best started in small portions, mixed into ground meat, eaten as pâté, or used once or twice weekly rather than treated like a large daily entrée. That is not because liver is weak. It is because it is strong. Heart is often easier for people because it behaves more like a dense working muscle and usually fits ordinary savory cooking more naturally. Kidney, spleen, marrow, and other organs can widen the range further, but they do not all need to appear at once for the pattern to become nutritionally meaningful. A modern diet does not need theatrical organ consumption. It needs repeated contact with more than one tissue type so nutrient coverage stops collapsing into muscle meat alone.

Preparation matters here because practicality is partly digestive and partly psychological. Organs that are cooked badly often fail twice. They taste harsher, and people conclude the food itself is the problem. Small portions, proper trimming, soaking when appropriate, pairing with familiar fats and seasonings, and using organs inside mixed preparations can lower friction without lowering the biological value. This is especially true for liver, where texture and mineral intensity can turn beginners away if the serving is too large or the cooking is careless. Integration works best when the food is made normal. Ground liver blended into beef, heart cut into stews or skewers, marrow used with roasted meat, or liver pâté eaten in modest amounts all accomplish the same deeper goal. They return metabolically active tissues to the diet without demanding that every meal feel like a challenge.

The final practical point is restraint through understanding, not fear. Organs are dense enough that more is not automatically better. Liver in particular should be respected as concentrated regulatory nutrition, not treated like a limitless health food. The body benefits from the density, but the density is the reason moderation makes sense. Small repeated inclusion usually does more good than erratic excess. This is especially important for people with unusual sensitivity, children, or pregnancy-related concerns, where very high retinol exposure from liver may need more caution. The practical modern solution is therefore simple. Build the diet on muscle meat, eggs, dairy, and other broadly usable animal foods. Add organs regularly in smaller amounts. Let tissue diversity widen micronutrient coverage without turning the menu into a performance. That is how nose-to-tail eating becomes sustainable. It stops being an ideology and starts becoming ordinary food again.

Part VI

Energy Metabolism and Metabolic Stability

Chapter 20

Why Cells Need Energy

Cells need energy because nothing in living tissue is allowed to stay still for long. Membranes have to hold electrical gradients. Ion pumps have to move sodium, potassium, calcium, and hydrogen against concentration differences. Proteins have to be synthesized, folded, transported, repaired, and degraded. Muscle has to contract. Glands have to secrete. Neurons have to fire. The intestine has to absorb. The liver has to sort, convert, and detoxify. None of that runs on abstract calories. It runs on adenosine triphosphate, or ATP, the immediate energy currency the cell can spend on demand. ATP is not stored in massive bulk the way fat is stored in adipose tissue. The cell keeps only a small working supply because ATP is made to be turned over rapidly. It is a short-range spending molecule, not a long-term reserve. This is why metabolism has to run continuously. The body cannot eat once, bank ATP for a month, and slowly draw it down. It has to keep converting food, oxygen, and stored fuel into fresh ATP moment by moment because the machinery of life is consuming it moment by moment.

The reason ATP works as a universal currency is chemical. Its phosphate bonds carry transferable energy in a form enzymes can use directly. When ATP loses one phosphate and becomes adenosine diphosphate, or ADP, energy is released in a controlled packet that can be coupled to cellular work. A membrane pump can use it to move ions. A muscle fiber can use it to power contraction. A biosynthetic pathway can use it to assemble molecules that would not form spontaneously under ordinary cellular conditions. This coupling is one of the deepest organizing principles in biology. The cell does not do work by setting food on fire inside itself. It breaks food down through staged biochemical pathways and captures part of that released energy in ATP so the energy can be delivered to the exact process that needs it. That is the crucial distinction. ATP turns raw nutrient energy into spendable biological action.

This also explains why food type matters metabolically. The body is not trying to maximize heat. It is trying to maintain ATP production with enough stability, enough substrate flexibility, and enough structural support that tissues can keep functioning without constant crisis. Glucose can be turned into ATP relatively quickly. Fatty acids can yield large amounts of ATP through slower oxidative metabolism. Amino acids can contribute when needed, though burning them as fuel is not their primary value because they are also the body's structural substrate. Vitamins and minerals matter here because many of the enzymes that generate ATP depend on them as cofactors. Oxygen matters because oxidative phosphorylation, the main mitochondrial process that generates most ATP, depends on a functioning electron transport chain. So ATP sits at the center of the whole picture. Food, oxygen, mitochondria, enzymes, membranes, and cofactors all converge on the same question. Can the cell keep producing enough spendable energy to maintain order.

The deeper point is that ATP makes metabolic stability measurable in the right place. A person may consume plenty of calories and still produce unstable energy if the incoming food creates poor substrate handling, weak nutrient support, or disordered signaling. The body may have fuel available and still struggle at the cellular level if glucose control is erratic, mitochondrial function is compromised, or the diet keeps supplying energy without enough of the structural and regulatory materials required to convert that energy cleanly into ATP. This is why "energy" in ordinary conversation is often misleading. What people feel as stable or unstable energy is really the downstream result of how well cells are being supplied, how efficiently ATP is being produced, and how calm or chaotic the larger hormonal and fuel-partitioning environment has become. ATP is universal because every cell depends on it. The quality of life inside the organism depends on how steadily it can be made.

Why Life Depends on Continuous Energy Turnover

Life depends on continuous energy turnover because the body is not a structure that gets built once and then sits there passively. It is a moving system held together by constant work. Membranes are always leaking ions and have to keep restoring gradients. Proteins are always being folded, repaired, degraded, and replaced. Muscles are always maintaining tone even at rest. The heart is always contracting. The brain is always firing, signaling, sorting, and suppressing noise. The liver is always processing incoming nutrients, packaging lipids, converting amino acids, managing glucose, and detoxifying compounds that cannot be left loose in circulation. The kidney is always filtering plasma and reclaiming what should not be lost. Even stillness is expensive. A resting body is not inactive. It is a body spending energy continuously to keep organized chemistry from falling apart.

That is why ATP, adenosine triphosphate, cannot be thought of as a reserve tank. It is more like a rapidly spent operating currency. Cells keep only a small immediate supply because ATP is made to be used quickly and regenerated constantly. Once ATP donates a phosphate and becomes adenosine diphosphate, or ADP, the cell has to rebuild it again through glycolysis, fatty acid oxidation, and mitochondrial oxidative phosphorylation. This rebuilding never stops because the work never stops. Ion pumps in the membrane are using ATP now. Protein synthesis is using ATP now. Vesicles are being transported now. Calcium is being moved now. A cell that stops turning energy over does not become relaxed. It begins losing gradients, losing structure, losing selective transport, and losing control of its internal environment. Death at the cellular level is not mainly the absence of calories. It is the failure to sustain organized energy flow.

This continuous turnover also explains why fuel stability matters more than raw intake. The body can have food around it and still struggle if that food is not being turned into usable cellular energy cleanly enough. A person can eat enough calories and still feel unstable because the problem is not gross energy presence. The problem is whether nutrients are being absorbed, partitioned, and oxidized in a way that keeps ATP production steady across time. Rapid glucose spikes followed by sharp containment can create a very different experience from slower fat-based energy delivery paired with adequate protein. Both may contribute energy. The rate, signaling environment, and durability of that contribution are different. Since cells are not waiting for the next meal to begin spending energy, the quality of turnover matters. A body running on unstable delivery keeps having to solve urgency. A body receiving steadier substrate can maintain order with less strain.

Continuous energy turnover is also why micronutrients matter so much. ATP is not made by calories alone. It is made by enzyme systems that depend on magnesium, iron, copper, riboflavin, niacin, thiamine, and many other cofactors. Oxygen delivery matters. Thyroid signaling matters. Membrane integrity matters. Mitochondrial structure matters. The body does not convert food into life through one simple reaction. It runs a layered energy economy that has to remain intact from digestion to circulation to cellular uptake to mitochondrial function. If any part of that chain weakens, the organism may still be alive, but it feels the weakening as fatigue, poor recovery, unstable focus, weaker temperature regulation, or reduced resilience under stress. The energy problem is never just about how much fuel entered. It is about whether turnover can continue at the pace life requires.

So life depends on continuous energy turnover because living order is not self-maintaining. It has to be paid for continuously. Every heartbeat, every nerve impulse, every absorbed nutrient, every repaired membrane, every filtered molecule, every maintained gradient is a fresh energy event. The body survives only because it keeps turning fuel into spendable work without interruption. That is the real metabolic standard. Not how much energy is theoretically present, but whether the organism can keep converting it into organized function minute after minute without falling into disorder.

The Difference Between Food Energy and Usable Cellular Energy

Food energy is what a food potentially contains. Usable cellular energy is what the body actually turns into spendable work inside living tissue. Those are not the same thing. A food can enter the mouth carrying measurable caloric value and still fail to provide stable, efficient energy at the cellular level if digestion is poor, absorption is incomplete, transport is disordered, hormonal signaling is unstable, or mitochondrial metabolism lacks the cofactors and conditions required to convert substrate into adenosine triphosphate, or ATP. This is where most shallow nutrition language collapses. It treats the presence of energy in food as though it were equivalent to energy available to the organism. But the body is not a bomb calorimeter. It does not burn food in one step and call the result metabolism. It has to dismantle the food, absorb the useful parts, route them through blood, sort them through the liver, deliver them into cells, and then run them through layered biochemical systems before any of that potential energy becomes usable biological currency.

Digestion is the first break in the chain between food energy and cellular energy. A meal may contain protein, fat, and carbohydrate on paper, but until stomach acid denatures the proteins, bile emulsifies the fats, pancreatic enzymes hydrolyze the major macronutrients, and the intestine moves the resulting fragments across its absorptive surface, the cell still has nothing to spend. Even after absorption, the story is not finished. Glucose entering the bloodstream is not yet ATP. Fatty acids carried in chylomicrons are not yet ATP. Amino acids entering portal blood are not yet ATP. They are substrates. They still have to be partitioned, stored, released, oxidized, or incorporated into other pathways according to the body's current needs. A person can therefore be eating plenty of food and still producing weak energy if the chain from ingestion to oxidation is impaired or unstable.

The mitochondrion is where this distinction becomes impossible to ignore. Cells do not use calories directly. They use ATP, and most ATP is generated by mitochondrial oxidative phosphorylation, the process in which electrons derived from glucose, fatty acids, or in some cases amino acids move through the electron transport chain to drive ATP synthesis. That process depends on oxygen, intact membranes, functional enzymes, and a long list of micronutrient cofactors. Magnesium is needed throughout ATP biology. Iron and copper are central to electron transport. Riboflavin and niacin contribute electron-carrying forms. Thiamine is needed for key entry points into oxidative metabolism. The cell can therefore be surrounded by theoretical food energy and still struggle to generate usable energy if the metabolic machinery is underpowered. This is why nutrient density matters so much more than calorie language suggests. The body does not only need fuel. It needs the means to convert fuel into ATP cleanly and repeatedly.

Hormonal stability changes the same relationship. A meal built around refined carbohydrate may create a rapid rise in blood glucose and a rapid rise in insulin, which means plenty of fuel is present for a moment, but the delivery is abrupt and often short-lived. A meal built around protein and fat tends to produce slower nutrient entry and steadier post-meal fuel access. The caloric value of those meals may overlap. Their cellular energy experience does not. One can create volatility, repeated hunger, and the sense of being fed but unstable. The other can create steadier ATP supply because the substrate enters more gradually and the endocrine environment is less chaotic. Food energy is therefore only raw potential. Usable cellular energy depends on timing, digestion, absorption, transport, hormonal handling, and mitochondrial competence.

This is why people can feel tired, unstable, or hungry again soon after eating meals that were calorically sufficient. The food solved the arithmetic problem and failed the biological one. It entered the body as energy potential but did not become durable cellular energy with enough efficiency to support stable function. That is the real difference. Food energy belongs to the meal. Usable cellular energy belongs to the cell. Between the two sits the entire machinery of physiology.

Why Metabolism Is Controlled Release, Not Combustion

Metabolism is often described with language borrowed from fire. Burn calories. Burn fat. Burn sugar. Burn more than you eat. That language survives because it captures one narrow truth, nutrients can be oxidized, and oxidation releases energy. But it also distorts the event so badly that people begin picturing the body as a furnace with preferences. It is not. Combustion is rapid, indiscriminate oxidation that converts fuel into heat in one violent step. Metabolism is staged, enzyme-governed, tissue-specific release. It takes stored chemical energy apart in small controlled transfers, captures part of that energy in forms the cell can actually use, and only then allows work to happen. Food does not enter a flame inside the body. It enters a digestive tract, then blood, then cells, then mitochondria, and at each stage the organism decides what fraction of the incoming substrate will be stored, released, oxidized, rebuilt into tissue, or cleared. Heat is produced along the way, yes, but heat is a byproduct of regulated life, not the central mechanism.

The difference becomes obvious as soon as glucose enters a cell. The body does not ignite glucose and harvest the fire. It moves glucose through glycolysis, a stepwise pathway in which enzymes split and rearrange the molecule through a sequence of controlled reactions. Small amounts of adenosine triphosphate, or ATP, are captured. Reducing equivalents are transferred into nicotinamide adenine dinucleotide, or NADH. Pyruvate is produced and then either reduced to lactate under certain conditions or moved into the mitochondrion and converted into acetyl-CoA. From there the citric acid cycle strips electrons in an organized pattern and feeds them into the electron transport chain, where a proton gradient is built across the inner mitochondrial membrane. Only then does ATP synthase use that gradient to generate larger amounts of ATP. This is not combustion. This is regulated disassembly with energy capture at each stage. The body is breaking a molecule down slowly enough to keep the released energy useful instead of destructive.

Fat oxidation follows the same logic. A fatty acid is not torched. It is activated, transported into the mitochondrion when needed, and then processed through beta-oxidation, a repeated cycle that clips off two-carbon units as acetyl-CoA while generating NADH and flavin adenine dinucleotide, or FADH2. Those products then feed the same deeper mitochondrial machinery that produces ATP. Again, the point is control. The body is releasing energy in packets that can be transferred into ATP production, not dumping all of the potential energy at once as heat. If metabolism worked like true combustion, cells would destroy themselves. Proteins would denature indiscriminately, membranes would fail, and useful gradients would collapse. Life depends on preventing exactly that kind of chemical chaos. The cell needs energy, but it needs it at the right rate, in the right place, and in a spendable form.

This is why enzymes matter so much. Enzymes lower activation energy and channel molecules through specific reactions rather than letting them react randomly. They decide which bond is altered, which intermediate is formed, which cofactor accepts electrons, which substrate proceeds, and which route is blocked. Hormones then regulate the larger traffic pattern. Insulin, glucagon, cortisol, thyroid hormone, epinephrine, and others determine whether fuel is stored, released, or oxidized. The liver decides whether incoming substrate becomes glycogen, ketones, triglyceride, glucose, or urea. Adipose tissue decides whether fat is being stored or liberated. Muscle decides whether fuel is burned locally or glycogen is conserved. None of that resembles a furnace. A furnace does not sort, prioritize, and redirect. The body does. Metabolism is therefore not just oxidation. It is oxidation placed under governance.

The phrase controlled release also explains why food quality changes metabolic experience so much. A rapidly absorbed refined carbohydrate can deliver glucose into circulation in a way that forces fast hormonal containment. A protein-and-fat meal arrives more slowly, triggers different digestive programs, and supplies substrate on a longer timeline. The calories may be discussed as equal in crude energy terms, but the release pattern is not equal, and the release pattern is what cells actually live inside. One meal creates urgency. Another creates steadier access. One makes the body contain fuel aggressively. Another allows fuel to enter and be used more gradually. Metabolism is not just about what is present. It is about how quickly the system has to deal with what is present and what regulatory cost that timing imposes.

So metabolism is controlled release, not combustion, because life cannot survive on raw oxidation alone. It needs captured energy, timed delivery, selective routing, and cellular order. The body does not burn food the way fire burns wood. It dismantles nutrients through layers of enzymatic control and converts their energy into ATP, gradients, motion, transport, repair, and signaling. Fire destroys its fuel to produce heat. Metabolism extracts usable work while keeping the structure alive.

Chapter 21

Glycolysis and Glucose Handling

Glycolysis is the body's fast-entry pathway for glucose. When carbohydrate is digested into glucose and that glucose enters circulation, cells can pull it inward and begin extracting energy from it almost immediately through a ten-step sequence in the cytoplasm called glycolysis. Cytoplasm is the fluid interior of the cell outside the mitochondria. This matters because glycolysis does not require the full slower machinery of fat digestion, bile release, micelle formation, lymphatic transport, and gradual fatty acid delivery. Glucose can appear in blood quickly, cross into cells quickly, and be broken down quickly. That is why carbohydrate often feels like immediate energy. The body is not imagining it. Glycolysis is built for fast access. It takes a six-carbon glucose molecule, rearranges and splits it, and ends with two three-carbon molecules called pyruvate while capturing a small amount of adenosine triphosphate, or ATP, and reducing power in the form of nicotinamide adenine dinucleotide, or NADH. This is not the cell's deepest energy pathway, but it is its quickest opening move.

The speed comes with limits. Glycolysis produces ATP quickly, but not in large yield compared with full mitochondrial oxidation. It is useful when energy needs to appear fast, when oxygen handling is limited, or when a tissue has high short-term glucose demand. Red blood cells rely on it heavily because they have no mitochondria. Fast-twitch muscle fibers use it aggressively during intense effort when the demand for ATP outruns what slower oxidative systems can supply moment to moment. The brain can use glucose readily because it is continuously active and tightly defended metabolically. But glycolysis is not a complete nutritional story. By itself it is a front-end extraction system, not a final answer to long-duration energy needs. The pyruvate it produces still has to go somewhere. Under lower-oxygen or high-demand conditions it may be reduced to lactate so glycolysis can keep running. Under more stable conditions it can enter the mitochondrion, become acetyl-CoA, and feed the citric acid cycle for much larger ATP production. So glycolysis is fast partly because it begins before the deeper machinery has fully taken over.

This is why glucose handling is so influential metabolically. A meal rich in refined carbohydrate can generate a rapid glucose influx that makes glycolysis available almost immediately across many tissues. That sounds useful, and in narrow contexts it is. But a fast-entry fuel also creates a fast regulatory problem. Blood glucose cannot be allowed to drift upward indefinitely, so insulin rises to contain it, direct it into cells, promote glycogen formation where there is room, and push the body toward fed-state handling. Glycolysis therefore sits close to endocrine control. The faster glucose arrives, the more aggressively the body may need to respond. A whole food carbohydrate embedded in tougher structure enters this pathway more gradually. A refined starch or sugar load can hit it hard and early. The pathway is the same. The tempo is different, and tempo changes the metabolic experience.

This is why glycolysis is best understood as short-term rapid energy extraction rather than as the body's preferred total fuel strategy. It is excellent at solving immediate demand. It is less suited to carrying the entire organism calmly for long intervals when meals are built around fast carbohydrate and weak structural value. If glucose keeps arriving rapidly, glycolysis keeps opening the same short-range door, and the body keeps needing insulin, storage decisions, and repeated fuel management to keep things stable. That can work. It is not free. Stable metabolism depends on more than having a rapid pathway available. It depends on whether the organism is being forced to live inside that pathway too often. Glycolysis is a useful tool. It becomes a problem when fast extraction turns into the dominant rhythm of feeding.

Pyruvate, Lactate, and the Early Stages of Glucose Metabolism

Once glucose enters the cell and glycolysis begins, the molecule is not being burned all at once. It is being dismantled in stages, and one of the key early end points of that staged breakdown is pyruvate. Glycolysis takes one six-carbon glucose molecule and converts it into two three-carbon pyruvate molecules while capturing a small amount of ATP and reducing equivalents in the form of NADH. Pyruvate is important because it sits at a metabolic fork. It is not waste. It is a decision point. What happens next depends on oxygen availability, mitochondrial capacity, the speed of ATP demand, and the larger metabolic state of the cell. This is one reason early glucose metabolism matters so much. The body is not simply extracting energy. It is deciding how urgently that energy is needed and how much of the deeper oxidative machinery can be engaged.

When oxygen delivery and mitochondrial function are adequate, pyruvate is usually transported into the mitochondrion and converted into acetyl-CoA by the pyruvate dehydrogenase complex, an enzyme system that links glycolysis to deeper oxidative metabolism. Acetyl-CoA then enters the citric acid cycle, where much more energy can be extracted through controlled oxidation and ultimately turned into ATP by oxidative phosphorylation. This is the higher-yield path. But it is slower and more dependent on intact mitochondrial function, oxygen supply, and micronutrient cofactors. So even though glucose can begin producing ATP quickly through glycolysis alone, the full energetic value of glucose depends on whether pyruvate can move forward into mitochondrial metabolism. Early glucose handling is therefore not just about speed. It is about whether fast extraction can transition cleanly into efficient deeper oxidation.

Lactate enters the picture when that forward movement is limited or when ATP demand is rising faster than mitochondrial processing can keep up. In those conditions pyruvate is reduced to lactate by lactate dehydrogenase. This step regenerates NAD+, which glycolysis needs in order to continue. That point is often missed. Lactate production is not just a sign of failure or metabolic collapse. It is part of how the cell keeps short-term ATP generation running when rapid glycolytic flux outpaces the slower downstream oxidative systems. The body is buying time. It is keeping glucose breakdown moving even when pyruvate cannot be fed into mitochondria quickly enough. That is why lactate rises during intense exercise, stress states, and other conditions where demand is immediate. Glycolysis is still doing its job. It is simply doing it under constrained conditions.

The older story that lactate is merely toxic waste or the singular cause of muscle soreness is too crude. Lactate is a real metabolic intermediate. It can leave one tissue and be used elsewhere. The liver can convert it back into glucose through gluconeogenesis in the Cori cycle. The heart and some oxidative tissues can use lactate directly as fuel under the right conditions. What matters here is that lactate formation marks a shift in how glucose is being handled. The cell is leaning harder on rapid short-range extraction and temporarily relying less on full mitochondrial oxidation. That can be adaptive in the moment. It is not the same thing as a calm, durable energy strategy for the organism as a whole.

This is why pyruvate and lactate reveal so much about glucose metabolism early in the sequence. Glucose enters fast, glycolysis produces ATP fast, pyruvate appears, and then the cell has to choose between deeper oxidation and temporary reduction to lactate depending on conditions. That makes carbohydrate metabolism powerful and useful, but also inherently tied to regulation, timing, and demand. A body living on rapid repeated glucose entry is repeatedly asking cells to solve short-term fuel problems. Sometimes that is appropriate. Sometimes it becomes the dominant metabolic rhythm and starts creating instability. Pyruvate and lactate are the first visible markers of that rhythm. They show whether glucose is moving calmly into oxidative metabolism or being handled in a more urgent and limited way.

Why Carbohydrate Energy Is Fast but Limited

Carbohydrate energy is fast because glucose can be moved into circulation and into cells with relatively little delay compared with fat. Starch is broken down into absorbable sugars. Those sugars enter portal blood quickly. Insulin rises to direct glucose into tissues, and glycolysis can begin extracting ATP in the cytoplasm almost immediately. That is the advantage. The body can solve an urgent fuel problem quickly. A rapidly contracting muscle, a stressed organism, or any state that needs immediate glucose access can use this pathway because it does not require bile-driven fat digestion, lymphatic transport, or the slower sequence that makes dietary fat available. Glucose can be delivered and processed in a hurry. That is why carbohydrate feels like quick energy. The chemistry is built for rapid entry and rapid early extraction.

The same feature that makes it fast also makes it limited. Glucose is tightly regulated because too much circulating in blood is dangerous and too little is also dangerous. The body cannot let it drift widely. That means carbohydrate energy depends on active hormonal containment from the start. Insulin has to rise, tissues have to take glucose in, glycogen stores in liver and muscle can only hold so much, and once those storage limits are approached the body is forced into a different set of decisions. Use it now. Store it as glycogen if there is room. Convert excess through hepatic pathways if the load keeps coming. This is not how long-range fuel behaves. A long-range fuel can be carried in large reserve without needing to remain within a narrow circulating window. Glucose cannot. It is useful precisely because it is tightly managed, but that same tight management is what makes it a shorter-range and less forgiving energy source.

The storage side proves the point. Glycogen, the storage form of glucose in liver and muscle, is useful but limited. It is stored with water, which means it is bulky relative to fat. The body cannot carry large multi-day energy reserves as glycogen the way it can as adipose fat. Muscle glycogen is also local. It is held for the muscle that stored it, not as a freely shared systemic reserve. Liver glycogen helps stabilize blood glucose, but its capacity is still modest. Once glycogen falls, the body has to shift. It can mobilize fat, produce ketones, and make glucose through gluconeogenesis, the endogenous production of glucose from non-carbohydrate substrates. That shift is not a metabolic defect. It is evidence that carbohydrate was never designed to be the only durable fuel system. It is a fast-access system sitting inside a larger organism built with backup and longer-range energy strategies.

Carbohydrate energy is also limited by the kind of appetite pattern it can create when delivered in refined form. A fast glucose rise is often followed by a faster endocrine response and, depending on meal composition and metabolic condition, a quicker drop in available circulating fuel. If the meal was low in protein and weak in fat, the person may feel the transition more sharply because the body received rapid substrate without much structural completion or long-duration buffering. This is why carbohydrate-heavy meals can produce a sense of quick energy and then quick appetite, especially when they come from refined flour, sugar, or other low-resistance forms. The pathway is doing what it was built to do. It is solving the short-term problem. It is simply not solving the full meal in a durable way.

That is the deeper meaning of fast but limited. Carbohydrate is effective at rapid ATP support, rapid glucose availability, and urgent metabolic response. It is less effective as a calm long-range strategy when it becomes the dominant rhythm of feeding and is repeatedly delivered in refined forms that keep the body solving the same short-term fuel problem again and again. The body can use carbohydrate well. It does not need to pretend carbohydrate is a stable unlimited energy base in order to do so. The speed is real. The limits are real too.

How Repeated Glucose-Heavy Feeding Shapes the Metabolic Environment

Repeated glucose-heavy feeding changes the metabolic environment by training the body to expect rapid fuel delivery over and over again, then forcing it to build its regulatory habits around that pattern. Every glucose-heavy meal or snack sends a similar message. Fast substrate is arriving. Blood sugar must be contained. Insulin must rise. Tissues must take in glucose, glycogen must be replenished where there is room, and excess must be pushed into other storage pathways if the incoming load keeps exceeding immediate demand. One such event is not the issue. The problem is repetition. When the body is exposed to this pattern several times a day, day after day, it stops dealing with glucose as an occasional fast fuel and starts living inside a metabolic climate shaped by frequent insulin signaling, repeated swings in available circulating fuel, and shorter intervals between energy peaks and energy decline. The organism becomes less dependent on mobilizing stored fat between meals because fast glucose keeps arriving before that shift has to happen fully. In practical terms, the body gets better at handling repeated intake and worse at living calmly between intakes.

This matters because the metabolic environment is not just the blood glucose number after one meal. It is the total hormonal and fuel-partitioning context the tissues are forced to inhabit over time. Frequent glucose-heavy feeding keeps insulin elevated more often, keeps glycogen turnover more active, and keeps the liver and muscle in a more continuous fed-state posture. Lipolysis, the release of stored fat from adipose tissue, is suppressed more regularly because the body is being told that incoming fuel is already present and should be used or stored first. Appetite can become more unstable because the meal solved the short-term fuel problem quickly without always solving the structural one. If protein is weak and fat is low, the person may cycle back into hunger sooner even though the body has already been through another large glucose event. That repeated cycle begins to shape perception as well as physiology. Energy starts to feel normal only when food is recent. The space between meals feels less calm because the body has been taught to expect another quick delivery rather than to rely more deeply on slower substrate release.

The liver is one of the main organs that absorbs this pressure. With repeated glucose-heavy feeding, especially when fructose and refined starch are part of the pattern, the liver is repeatedly asked to handle incoming carbohydrate, replenish glycogen, convert excess substrate, and maintain blood glucose control between meals. That does not make carbohydrate uniquely toxic in all contexts. It means carbohydrate-heavy eating has a distinct metabolic cost when it becomes the dominant rhythm of the diet. The liver becomes more central to constant traffic control. The pancreas becomes more central to constant insulin release. Peripheral tissues are exposed to the same repeated instruction that glucose is abundant now and must be managed now. Over time, the body is living in a more compressed energy pattern, one built around containment and redistribution rather than around broader flexibility in fuel selection.

This repeated environment can also change what kind of appetite and energy the person experiences as normal. Meals rich in refined carbohydrate often deliver fast energy with weaker satiety than meals built around substantial protein and fat. If that pattern is repeated often enough, the person may stop noticing that the system has become dependent on frequent refeeding to maintain stable mood and function. Cravings rise more easily. Midday slumps become familiar. Hunger appears sooner. The person may interpret this as normal metabolism or personal weakness, but much of it is simply the downstream behavior of a body living inside a glucose-dominant rhythm. The metabolic environment has been trained toward urgency. A system repeatedly fed for speed begins to organize around speed.

Chapter 22

Fat Oxidation and Long-Duration Energy

Fatty acids function as long-range fuel because the body can store them densely, release them gradually, and oxidize them over extended periods without needing the same constant containment that glucose requires. A fatty acid is a long hydrocarbon chain, a highly reduced molecule carrying substantial chemical energy in its carbon-hydrogen bonds. Once liberated from triglycerides and made available to tissues, that chain can be moved into mitochondria and broken down step by step through beta-oxidation, producing acetyl-CoA, NADH, and FADH2, the reduced cofactors that later feed the electron transport chain for ATP production. This is not fast emergency energy. It is slower, deeper energy extraction built for duration. The body is not solving a short spike. It is drawing from a substrate meant to sustain work over time.

That long-range character begins before oxidation even starts. Dietary fat is digested more slowly than refined carbohydrate. It leaves the stomach more slowly, depends on bile for emulsification, requires lipase for hydrolysis, and enters circulation through lymphatic transport as chylomicrons rather than appearing rapidly in portal blood as glucose does. Stored body fat behaves similarly in principle. It is mobilized when needed through lipolysis, released as free fatty acids, carried on albumin in the bloodstream, and taken up by tissues that can oxidize it. The whole system is built around paced release rather than immediate flood. That matters because a fuel that enters and leaves the active pool more gradually changes how the organism experiences energy. The body is less dependent on repeated external feeding when it can rely more confidently on fatty acid delivery between meals.

Fatty acids are also long-range fuel because the storage system built around them is large. Glycogen reserves are limited and stored with water. Fat reserves are compact and energy dense. The body can carry substantial amounts of potential fuel in adipose tissue without the bulk penalty that would come with storing the same energy as carbohydrate. This is not a small design detail. It tells you what kind of substrate the organism uses for durable reserve. If glucose is the quick-access drawer, fat is the warehouse. That does not make glucose unimportant. It clarifies hierarchy. The body can always use fast fuel when needed. It depends on fat to provide the deeper reserve that makes endurance, fasting tolerance, and metabolic steadiness possible.

This is why fatty acid use often feels calmer than heavy reliance on repeated glucose feeding. A tissue oxidizing fatty acids is not waiting on the next rapid blood sugar rise in the same way. It is drawing from a substrate that can be supplied from the meal or from stored reserves through a slower and more continuous stream. That tends to reduce urgency. Energy becomes less about quick rescue and more about ongoing provision. In a body that digests and oxidizes fat well, this often shows up as longer satiety, less volatility between meals, and less dependence on frequent eating to maintain stable function. The fuel is not magical. It is simply entering metabolism on a timeline that better fits long-duration work.

So when fatty acids are described as long-range fuel, the point is not that they burn hotter or better in every imaginable context. The point is that their digestion, storage, mobilization, and oxidation all favor sustained delivery over rapid turnover. They are the substrate the body leans on when the question is not how to solve the next few minutes, but how to keep the organism running cleanly across the next several hours.

Mitochondrial Oxidation and Sustained ATP Production

Mitochondrial oxidation is where the body turns nutrient-derived substrate into durable cellular energy rather than short-lived metabolic relief. Glycolysis can extract a small amount of adenosine triphosphate, or ATP, quickly in the cytoplasm, but that is only the front edge of energy metabolism. Sustained ATP production depends on what happens after that. Fatty acids broken down through beta-oxidation and pyruvate derived from glucose both converge on acetyl-CoA, which enters the mitochondrion and feeds the citric acid cycle. There, carbon fragments are progressively stripped for electrons, and those electrons are transferred into NADH and FADH2, the reduced carriers that deliver them to the electron transport chain. This is the deeper engine. The cell is no longer taking quick withdrawals from an easily accessed fuel pathway. It is moving substrate into the machinery built for higher-yield, longer-duration energy production.

The inner mitochondrial membrane is where this becomes real. The electron transport chain passes electrons from one protein complex to the next in a controlled sequence, and the energy released during that transfer is used to pump protons across the membrane. That creates an electrochemical gradient, a difference in charge and proton concentration across the membrane that functions like stored potential energy. ATP synthase then uses that gradient to turn adenosine diphosphate, or ADP, back into ATP. This is not a side detail in metabolism. It is the main way aerobic tissues stay powered. Muscle at rest, heart tissue, liver, kidneys, much of the brain, all depend heavily on this system because it can keep generating ATP over time as long as oxygen, substrate, intact membrane function, and the necessary cofactors are available. The mitochondrion is not burning fuel in bulk. It is harvesting electrons, building gradients, and converting that gradient into spendable energy with remarkable control.

This is why fat oxidation supports sustained energy so well. A fatty acid is a long carbon chain, and each round of beta-oxidation produces more acetyl-CoA, more NADH, and more FADH2, which means more input into the electron transport chain and more opportunity for ATP generation. The process is slower than rapid glycolytic flux, but it is far more suited to endurance. A tissue oxidizing fat efficiently can keep drawing ATP from a substrate that is dense, abundant, and available through a steadier supply line. That changes the character of energy. Instead of repeated short-term glucose surges followed by repeated containment and renewed hunger, the body can rely more on prolonged substrate flow through oxidative metabolism. The result is often experienced as steadier output, less urgency, and less dependence on constant feeding. The cell is not being rescued repeatedly. It is being supplied.

Sustained ATP production also depends on more than fuel alone. Mitochondria require oxygen as the final electron acceptor. They require iron and copper inside the electron transport chain. They require riboflavin and niacin to form FAD and NAD. They require magnesium throughout ATP biology. They require intact membranes, reasonable redox balance, and a cellular environment not constantly destabilized by overnutrition, undernutrition, inflammation, or repeated metabolic whiplash. This is why a person can eat enough calories and still produce poor energy. The issue may not be gross fuel shortage. It may be weak mitochondrial throughput. Food energy only becomes useful at this level if the oxidative machinery can actually turn substrate into ATP with enough efficiency to support the cell's ongoing work.

That is why mitochondrial oxidation sits at the center of metabolic stability. The body is not trying merely to get through the next hour. It is trying to keep ATP production running continuously across tissues that cannot afford interruption. Fast fuel can solve urgency. Mitochondrial oxidation solves continuity. It is the difference between temporary access and durable supply, between metabolic noise and sustained cellular work.

Why Fat-Based Metabolism Is Slower and Steadier

Fat-based metabolism is slower and steadier because the body cannot move fat from plate to ATP with the same speed it uses for glucose. Every stage takes longer. Dietary fat leaves the stomach more slowly. It has to be emulsified by bile because it does not mix with the watery contents of the intestine. Pancreatic lipase has to hydrolyze triglycerides into fatty acids and monoglycerides. Those lipid fragments have to be organized into micelles, absorbed into enterocytes, rebuilt into triglycerides, packaged into chylomicrons, and sent through lymphatic circulation before they even join the bloodstream in meaningful quantity. That route is slower by design. The body is not receiving a sudden wave of blood sugar that must be contained immediately. It is receiving a staged lipid supply that enters circulation more gradually and moves into tissues on a longer timeline. The chemistry forces patience, and that patience is part of why the energy feels different.

Once fatty acids reach the cell, the same pattern continues. They are not simply dropped into a fast cytoplasmic pathway the way glucose enters glycolysis. They must be activated, transported into the mitochondrion when appropriate, and then broken down through beta-oxidation into acetyl-CoA units that feed the citric acid cycle and oxidative phosphorylation. That process yields large amounts of ATP, but it is not built for urgency. It is built for duration. The body is using a denser fuel through a slower extraction system. This means fat-based metabolism tends to support a calmer energy state, one less dependent on repeated feeding and less vulnerable to the rapid rise-and-fall pattern that often follows heavy reliance on refined carbohydrate. The ATP arrives through a deeper oxidative process rather than through short-term glycolytic rescue.

The hormonal environment reflects the same difference. A glucose-heavy meal often produces a faster insulin event because blood glucose has to be managed quickly once it rises. A fat-rich meal, especially when paired with substantial protein, tends to slow gastric emptying, increase cholecystokinin and other satiety signals, and reduce the urgency of post-meal fuel handling. The body is not being told that a fast substrate flood has arrived and must be stored, burned, or contained now. It is being told that a slower fuel and structural meal is being processed over time. That changes appetite, energy, and the space between meals. A person relying more on fat oxidation is often less dependent on constant intake because the metabolic system is drawing from a fuel that enters slowly and can also be supplied steadily from body fat stores between meals.

This does not mean fat-based metabolism is inert or universally superior in every context. It means its tempo is different. Carbohydrate solves immediate demand well. Fat supports extended demand well. When metabolism leans more heavily on fat, the body generally spends less time living inside repeated glucose spikes, repeated insulin responses, and repeated short-interval hunger. It spends more time drawing from a slower substrate stream through mitochondrial oxidation. That is why fat-based metabolism feels steadier. Not because fat is magical, but because every major step, digestion, absorption, transport, mobilization, and oxidation, unfolds on a longer and more controlled timeline.

Why Higher-Fat Eating Can Shift Energy Stability

Higher-fat eating can shift energy stability because it changes both the timing of digestion and the dominant fuel environment the body is being asked to live in. A meal built around more fat and adequate protein does not enter the system like a glucose-heavy meal. It leaves the stomach more slowly, requires bile release and pancreatic lipase activity, moves through micelle formation and lymphatic transport, and delivers fuel over a longer interval. That slower digestive sequence changes what happens after the meal. The body is not being hit with the same rapid rise in blood glucose or the same urgent demand for insulin-mediated containment. Instead, nutrient delivery is stretched out, satiety tends to last longer, and the person is less likely to feel the sharp post-meal swing that often follows meals built around refined starch and sugar. The shift is mechanical before it is subjective. The fuel is arriving on a different timeline, so the energy pattern feels different.

This matters because metabolic instability is often a timing problem as much as a quantity problem. A person may be eating enough calories and still feel volatile if those calories keep arriving in forms that push rapid glucose entry, short-term glycolysis, repeated insulin release, and frequent return of hunger. In that state, energy tends to feel borrowed. It rises quickly, falls quickly, and has to be replaced quickly. Higher-fat eating changes that rhythm by giving the body more access to a slower substrate and by reducing dependence on repeated fast carbohydrate delivery. The body still uses glucose where needed. It does not become anti-glucose. But it spends less of the day trapped in urgent glucose handling and more of the day drawing from fatty acids delivered from the meal or released from adipose tissue between meals. That wider use of fat oxidation often feels like steadier energy because the organism is no longer solving the same short-range fuel problem over and over.

Protein strengthens this effect because higher-fat eating that is not paired with adequate protein can become heavy without becoming nutritionally decisive. When fat and protein rise together, the meal tends to become more biologically complete. Protein supplies amino acids for repair and stronger satiety signaling. Fat extends digestion and slows energy delivery. Together they often reduce the need to keep eating simply to stabilize mood and function. This is where higher-fat eating often changes appetite as well as energy. The person may notice less urgency around food, longer gaps between meals that feel natural rather than forced, and less dependence on snacks or quick carbohydrate rescue. The body is not only receiving a slower fuel. It is receiving a meal that is more likely to feel finished.

The shift can also expose weaknesses in digestion. A body coming from years of low-fat or glucose-heavy eating may not handle higher-fat intake smoothly at first if bile flow is poor, gallbladder contraction is weak, or pancreatic contribution is underpowered. In that case the person may mistake digestive difficulty for proof that higher-fat eating is inherently wrong for him. Often the more honest interpretation is that the digestive machinery for fat was underused, undertrained, or burdened. If liver, gallbladder, bile, pancreatic lipase, intestinal absorption, and lymphatic transport are functioning well, higher-fat eating often improves energy stability precisely because it gives the body a slower and more durable substrate. If those systems are compromised, the transition can feel rough until the digestive side is addressed.

So higher-fat eating can shift energy stability because it changes the entire fuel pattern of the day. Meals digest more slowly. Nutrients enter more gradually. Satiety lasts longer. Insulin urgency often falls. Fat oxidation becomes more relevant. Stored body fat becomes easier to access between meals rather than remaining functionally sidelined by repeated glucose-heavy feeding. None of this means every high-fat meal is automatically stabilizing or that context stops mattering. It means the body often becomes steadier when it is no longer being forced to run on rapid fuel turnover as its default rhythm. Higher-fat eating does not create energy out of nowhere. It changes the tempo of delivery, and the tempo is often what unstable metabolism was missing.

Chapter 23

Ketones, Metabolic Flexibility, and the Facultative Carnivore Engine

Ketone production begins when fat is no longer being treated mainly as stored backup or meal-associated energy, but as a primary substrate the body is actively converting into a transportable fuel. This happens in the liver. Fatty acids released from adipose tissue or absorbed from a fat-rich meal are taken up and moved into mitochondria, where beta-oxidation breaks them into repeated two-carbon units in the form of acetyl-CoA. Under ordinary mixed-feeding conditions, much of that acetyl-CoA can move through the citric acid cycle and be oxidized there. But when carbohydrate availability is lower, insulin is lower, glucagon is relatively higher, and hepatic glucose production is being maintained through gluconeogenesis, the liver begins routing some of that acetyl-CoA differently. Oxaloacetate, the four-carbon molecule that helps accept acetyl-CoA into the citric acid cycle, is being pulled toward glucose maintenance rather than sitting freely available for unlimited oxidation. The liver is still receiving a large stream of fat-derived acetyl-CoA, but the ordinary oxidative entry point has become relatively constrained. Ketogenesis is the solution. The liver condenses acetyl-CoA into ketone bodies, mainly acetoacetate and beta-hydroxybutyrate, which is technically not a true ketone by strict chemistry but is grouped with them because it behaves as part of the same fuel system. What was once local fat-derived substrate is now packaged into a circulating energy currency that other tissues can use.

This matters because long-chain fatty acids cannot simply replace glucose everywhere in the same direct way. Some tissues need glucose continuously, and the brain cannot rely on long-chain fatty acids as its main fuel because they do not cross the blood-brain barrier efficiently in meaningful amounts. Ketones solve that transport problem. They are water-soluble enough to move through blood without being packaged the way dietary fat is packaged in chylomicrons, and they can cross into tissues, including the brain, where they are converted back into acetyl-CoA and oxidized for ATP production. In practical terms, ketogenesis is the body's way of turning stored or incoming fat into a shareable fuel. The liver makes the ketones, but the liver does not use them heavily itself. It releases them outward. Heart, skeletal muscle, brain, and other tissues can then draw on them when the metabolic environment says carbohydrate is not the dominant incoming fuel. This is one reason ketones matter so much in a facultative carnivore framework. They make fat usable not only as a slow local fuel, but as a system-wide fuel that can reduce dependence on repeated glucose delivery.

Ketone production therefore signals a larger metabolic shift. The body is no longer organizing the day around constant external carbohydrate supply. It is drawing more confidently from fatty acids, converting part of that flux into ketones, and using those ketones to stabilize the space between meals. Hunger often changes here because the person is no longer depending on rapid glucose entry to feel normal. Energy often changes because the body is not being pushed through the same repeated pattern of fast absorption, insulin containment, and short-interval refueling. None of this means ketones are magic or that all ketosis is automatically beneficial regardless of context. It means ketogenesis is one of the body's built-in tools for extending the usefulness of fat beyond adipose storage and beyond slow local oxidation. It widens the fuel field. It gives the organism another way to remain powered when glucose intake falls and fat availability rises.

This is why ketone production from fat belongs at the center of metabolic flexibility rather than at the fringe of dietary ideology. A flexible organism needs more than one way to stay fed internally. It needs to manage glucose when glucose is present, oxidize fatty acids when fatty acids are available, and produce ketones when the conditions favor fat-derived long-range fuel. The facultative carnivore engine depends on that range. Protein supplies structural material. Fat supplies durable substrate. The liver then converts part of that fat into ketones when the broader hormonal and fuel environment calls for it. What changes is not only what the body is eating. What changes is what kind of internal energy economy the body is running. Ketone production marks the moment fat stops being merely stored potential and becomes an active circulating fuel for the whole organism.

Why the Brain Can Use More Than Glucose

The brain is often described as if it runs on glucose alone, but that statement is only partially true and becomes misleading the moment metabolism shifts away from constant carbohydrate supply. The brain certainly uses glucose, and some glucose requirement remains because certain cellular processes and supporting tissues still depend on it. But that is not the same as saying the brain is locked to glucose as its only serious fuel. It is not. When fat oxidation rises and the liver begins producing ketone bodies from fatty acids, the brain can take in those ketones and oxidize them for ATP production at substantial levels. This is one of the body's built-in solutions to a basic energy problem. Long-chain fatty acids do not cross the blood-brain barrier efficiently enough to serve as the brain's main direct fuel, but ketones do. The liver therefore converts part of the fat stream into a transportable form the brain can actually use.

This changes the whole picture of metabolic dependence. Under glucose-heavy feeding, the brain is supplied largely through circulating glucose, and that works because carbohydrate is arriving often enough and insulin-regulated handling is keeping blood glucose within a narrow range. When carbohydrate intake falls or meals are spaced further apart, the body does not simply allow brain energy to collapse. The liver increases gluconeogenesis, the endogenous production of glucose from non-carbohydrate substrates, and it increases ketogenesis, the production of ketone bodies from fatty acid-derived acetyl-CoA. Those ketones, mainly beta-hydroxybutyrate and acetoacetate, cross into the brain and are converted back into acetyl-CoA inside neural tissue, where they enter mitochondrial oxidation and support ATP production. In practical terms, the body begins sharing fat-derived energy with the brain through a different currency.

That matters because it means the brain is metabolically more flexible than modern nutrition language usually allows. The common story implies that frequent carbohydrate intake is required because the brain must be fed glucose continually from the outside. But the body does not leave such a critical organ dependent on constant meal-to-meal carbohydrate rescue. It preserves blood glucose where needed, yes, but it also creates a parallel fuel stream so the brain can draw heavily from ketones when the metabolic environment changes. This is not a starvation-only emergency trick. It is part of normal human fuel adaptability. The brain can shift a substantial share of its energy burden away from glucose when ketones are available in meaningful quantity, which reduces the total glucose that must be supplied at that moment.

The advantage of this is not only survival. It also changes the feel of energy. A brain depending more heavily on ketones is not waiting on repeated rapid glucose entry to remain powered. It is drawing from a substrate linked to fat availability and hepatic production, which tends to produce a steadier internal fuel pattern. That does not mean ketones are superior in every circumstance or that glucose becomes irrelevant. It means the brain has more than one serious fuel option, and that option becomes especially important when the body is not being fed frequent carbohydrate. This is one reason a facultative carnivore framework makes physiological sense. The body can maintain glucose where glucose is required while simultaneously reducing whole-body dependence on glucose as the dominant daily fuel.

So the claim that the brain can use more than glucose is not a clever exception to the rule. It is part of the rule. The brain remains glucose-dependent in part, but not glucose-exclusive in the deeper energetic sense. Ketones allow fat-derived energy to enter a tissue that cannot rely directly on long-chain fatty acids, and that widens the organism's entire metabolic range. The result is a brain that can remain powered even when carbohydrate intake is lower, meals are less frequent, and fat oxidation has become more central to the body's energy economy.

Fuel Switching Between Fed and Low-Carbohydrate States

Fuel switching is the body's ability to change what it is running on without losing control of energy production. In the fed state, especially after a carbohydrate-rich meal, glucose enters circulation, insulin rises, and tissues are told that incoming fuel is abundant now. Some of that glucose is oxidized immediately. Some is stored as glycogen in liver and muscle. Lipolysis, the release of stored fat from adipose tissue, is suppressed because the body has no reason to mobilize reserve fuel while fresh glucose is arriving and being distributed. This is a normal fed pattern. The body is not broken when it does this. It is responding to the chemistry of the meal. Fast substrate came in, so the organism shifts toward glucose handling, containment, storage where appropriate, and immediate use where demand exists.

A low-carbohydrate state changes that sequence because the external glucose stream becomes smaller and less frequent. Insulin falls relative to the fed carbohydrate state. Glucagon rises. Glycogen stores are drawn down instead of repeatedly topped off. The liver increases gluconeogenesis to maintain the portion of blood glucose still required by certain tissues, and adipose tissue begins releasing more fatty acids into circulation because the body now has to rely more on internal fuel mobilization. The liver takes up some of those fatty acids, oxidizes them, and begins converting part of that flux into ketone bodies when conditions favor ketogenesis. Muscle and other tissues increase their use of fatty acids directly. The brain, which cannot rely heavily on long-chain fatty acids themselves, begins using more ketones as they become available. This is fuel switching in practice. The body is not shutting down because carbohydrate fell. It is reorganizing which substrates are carrying the greater share of the load.

What makes this important is that the switch is hormonal and metabolic, not ideological. The body does not care whether the eater calls the pattern low-carb, carnivore, ketogenic, or anything else. It cares what is arriving through the intestine, what is absent, what glycogen status looks like, what insulin is signaling, and whether stored fuel needs to be mobilized. If carbohydrate is frequent and substantial, glucose handling dominates more of the day. If carbohydrate falls and protein and fat become more central, fat oxidation and ketone production rise to fill the space. Both states are part of human physiology. The deeper question is whether the person can move between them cleanly or whether he has become metabolically dependent on one narrow pattern of frequent glucose supply.

This is why metabolic flexibility matters so much. A flexible system can accept a carbohydrate meal and handle it without chaos, then later go hours without food and shift toward fatty acid use and ketone production without feeling metabolically trapped. An inflexible system often does the opposite. It handles the fed state poorly and handles the gap between meals poorly as well. Blood sugar feels unstable. Hunger arrives fast. Mood and focus become too dependent on the next glucose input. Stored fat exists, but access to it feels metabolically muffled because the body is not switching easily. In that state, the problem is not simply what fuel is available. The problem is that the transition between fuels has become weak.

A facultative carnivore framework depends on this switching ability because it places more of the day on the fat-oxidation side of the ledger while still preserving the body's ability to use glucose where needed. Protein supplies structure. Fat supplies the slower and larger fuel stream. The liver maintains glucose production for tissues that still require it and produces ketones to widen access to fat-derived energy. The person is no longer relying on constant carbohydrate entry to feel normal because the body has switched more confidently into a different internal energy economy. That does not mean glucose becomes unimportant. It means glucose stops being the only fuel the person feels capable of running on comfortably. Fuel switching is the mechanism that makes that possible.

Why Metabolic Flexibility Matters More Than Dietary Dogma

Metabolic flexibility matters more than dietary dogma because the body is not trying to defend a food philosophy. It is trying to remain powered under changing conditions without losing control of blood glucose, tissue repair, appetite, or access to stored fuel. A rigid dietary identity starts with rules and categories. Metabolic flexibility starts with the organism. It asks whether the body can use glucose when glucose is present, whether it can shift toward fatty acid oxidation when carbohydrate falls, whether it can produce ketones when needed, and whether it can do all of that without creating constant urgency, constant hunger, or constant metabolic confusion. That is a much deeper question than whether a person belongs to the low-carb camp, the high-carb camp, or the balanced-diet camp. The body does not win by picking a slogan. It wins by being able to move between fuel states cleanly while still protecting structural nutrition.

This is why a person can follow a dietary doctrine perfectly and still remain metabolically brittle. A high-carbohydrate eater may be dependent on frequent glucose input to feel normal, with energy and mood beginning to sag as soon as the next meal is delayed. A low-carbohydrate eater may lower glucose variability and rely more on fat oxidation, but if protein is weak, digestion is poor, or the pattern is treated as ideology instead of physiology, the result can still become narrow and unstable. Dogma tends to turn one useful metabolic condition into a total worldview. Flexibility keeps the hierarchy clearer. Glucose is useful. Fat oxidation is useful. Ketone production is useful. The important issue is not whether one of these pathways can be turned into a personality. The important issue is whether the body can access the right one when conditions change and whether the person is eating in a way that supports that range rather than shrinking it.

The organism needs this range because life does not present food in one fixed pattern. Meals vary. Activity varies. Stress varies. Sleep varies. Illness changes demand. A body that can only feel functional when fed frequent carbohydrate is not flexible. A body that cannot handle carbohydrate at all without obvious disruption is not flexible either. A flexible system can accept carbohydrate and manage it without extreme volatility, then move into longer gaps between meals and draw from fatty acids and ketones without panic. It can preserve blood glucose where glucose is still required while allowing much of the organism to shift toward slower fuel. That range matters more than dogma because it reflects actual resilience. It is the difference between a metabolism that must be propped up repeatedly and one that can regulate itself across changing conditions.

This is also why a facultative carnivore framework should not be confused with a brittle commandment. The point is not that every person must live in one fuel state at all times or that any deviation destroys the model. The point is that human physiology appears to function especially well when protein and fat form the structural and energetic base, because that pattern often improves satiety, stabilizes energy, and restores access to the slower fuel systems the body was built to use. But the strength of that framework is not that it creates a new doctrine. Its strength is that it tends to widen metabolic competence. The person becomes less dependent on fast fuel, more able to run between meals, and more able to judge food by biological fit instead of by dietary identity. That is the real goal. Not loyalty to a label, but a metabolism that can use the full range of its own machinery without becoming trapped in one narrow rhythm of feeding.

Part VII

Hunger, Satiety, and Why Modern Diets Destabilize Appetite

Chapter 24

Hunger Is a Signal Problem

Hunger is not just the absence of food. It is the body's running interpretation of whether the last meal was sufficient, how quickly it is being processed, what nutrients are entering circulation, and whether the endocrine signals generated by that meal are strong enough to shut intake down for a while. Satiety is therefore not a moral achievement and not a simple matter of stomach volume. It is a timed biochemical response built from digestion, absorption, and hormonal feedback. The body has to sense that meaningful material has arrived, not merely that something was swallowed. Protein, fat, and carbohydrate do not produce the same satiety pattern because they do not move through the digestive tract at the same speed and do not generate the same hormonal sequence. A meal that creates strong satiety usually does two things well. It slows the digestive event enough for the body to register it, and it delivers enough structural and energetic value to make that slowing mean something.

This is where satiety hormones come in. Cholecystokinin, or CCK, rises when protein and fat enter the small intestine and helps slow gastric emptying while also signaling gallbladder contraction and pancreatic secretion. Peptide YY rises further down the intestinal tract in response to nutrient exposure and helps suppress appetite after the meal. Glucagon-like peptide-1, or GLP-1, is released from intestinal cells as nutrients move through and contributes to insulin coordination, slower gastric emptying, and reduced hunger. Ghrelin, by contrast, tends to rise before meals and fall when feeding becomes biologically meaningful. These hormones do not work in isolation. They act as part of a timing network. The stomach stretches, yes, but stretch alone is weak if the meal empties quickly and fails to generate a strong nutrient signal downstream. Lasting satiety depends on the intestine confirming that real digestion is underway and that useful material is entering the system.

Digestive timing is therefore central. Protein-rich and fat-rich meals tend to stay in the stomach longer, require more acid, more enzymatic work, more bile coordination, and more time for nutrients to appear in circulation. That slower sequence gives the body a better chance to build a layered satiety response. The stomach is still working. Amino acids are rising. Fatty acids are being absorbed. CCK and peptide YY are active. The meal feels finished because the body is still interacting with it as nourishment. A refined carbohydrate meal often behaves differently. It may empty faster, raise blood glucose faster, provoke insulin faster, and produce a much shorter digestive arc. The person gets energy quickly, but the deeper satiety sequence may be weaker because structural input was low and the meal moved through the system too fast to create durable completion. Hunger then returns not because appetite is irrational, but because the digestive clock ran too quickly and the endocrine response was too thin.

This is why modern diets destabilize appetite so easily. They repeatedly give the body meals that are fast in reward and fast in glucose delivery, but weak in the slower hormonal signals that tell the organism it has been properly fed. Soft texture reduces chewing time. Refined carbohydrate speeds absorption. Weak protein lowers structural completion. Industrial fat can add energy density without necessarily restoring a clean satiety pattern when it is mixed into processed food built around sugar and starch. The eater is left with a meal that was highly stimulating and poorly finishing. Hunger becomes a signal problem because the signals themselves were disordered. Satiety hormones are part of the body's braking system, but they only work well when the meal gives them a real reason to engage.

Why Protein and Fat Tend to Shut Down Appetite More Effectively

Protein and fat tend to shut down appetite more effectively because they do more than occupy space in the stomach. They create a slower, denser, more biologically meaningful meal. Protein arrives as structural material the body actually needs, not just as fuel. Fat arrives as slower fuel, membrane substrate, and a major trigger for bile-dependent digestion. Together they force the digestive tract into a more deliberate sequence.

Gastric emptying slows. Acid secretion matters more. Cholecystokinin rises. Peptide YY rises. The intestine has more time to confirm that real nutrients are being processed and absorbed. That timing is part of why the meal feels more finished. The body is not just sensing bulk. It is sensing that amino acids and fatty acids are arriving in forms worth responding to.

Protein is especially powerful here because appetite does not only track calories. It also tracks unresolved structural demand. The body has to keep rebuilding enzymes, muscle proteins, gut lining cells, immune molecules, connective tissue, and transport proteins continuously. It cannot do that from carbohydrate alone, and it does not keep a large reserve pool of free amino acids waiting to be drawn down at will. When a meal provides enough digestible, complete protein, the bloodstream begins receiving amino acids that tell the organism something important. Building material is here. Repair can proceed. The meal is doing more than solving the next hour of energy. It is feeding the body at the level of maintenance. Appetite tends to quiet under those conditions because one of the deeper biological reasons for continued food-seeking has actually been addressed.

Fat strengthens the same effect through a different mechanism. It slows the meal mechanically and hormonally. Fat in the small intestine triggers bile release and cholecystokinin, slows gastric emptying, and extends the timeline of digestion so nutrients keep arriving over a longer window. That matters because a short fast meal and a long dense meal do not produce the same satiety pattern even when they contain the same calories. A meal built around protein and fat keeps the digestive tract occupied with real work. It prolongs contact between food and the hormonal systems that regulate appetite. It also reduces the need for immediate rapid glucose replacement because fat provides a slower fuel stream once digestion and absorption are underway. The eater is therefore less likely to feel that abrupt gap between initial fullness and renewed hunger that often follows carbohydrate-dominant meals.

This is where modern processed food fails so often. It can deliver plenty of energy while producing a much weaker satiety signal because the meal is soft, fast, glucose-heavy, and structurally thin. The body gets quick fuel, but little durable completion. Protein may be too low. Fat may be present, but trapped inside a hyper-palatable starch-sugar mixture that drives intake faster than satiety can build. The mouth is impressed. The gut is underconvinced. By contrast, a meal built from meat, eggs, dairy, or other substantial animal foods usually creates a stronger biological stop signal because the nutrients arriving are dense, digestively consequential, and relevant to what the body is trying to maintain. Appetite shuts down more effectively when the organism is no longer being asked to keep searching for what the meal failed to supply.

So the reason protein and fat reduce appetite more effectively is not that they are magic hunger suppressants. It is that they feed the body more honestly. They slow the digestive sequence, strengthen satiety hormones, provide structural material, and extend fuel delivery in a way that makes the meal feel complete rather than merely caloric. Hunger falls more reliably when the body has a real reason to stop asking.

Why Refined Carbohydrates Often Fail to Finish the Meal Biologically

Refined carbohydrates often fail to finish the meal biologically because they solve the fastest part of hunger and leave the deeper part untouched. They deliver glucose quickly, raise blood sugar quickly, and can create an immediate sense of energy or relief, but that rapid fuel delivery is not the same thing as nutritional completion. A refined carbohydrate food has usually been stripped of much of its original structure. Fiber barriers are reduced. Water content is often low relative to whole foods. Protein is usually weak or incomplete. Fat, if present, is often added back in processed form rather than arriving as part of a coherent nutrient package. What reaches the body, then, is a meal designed for speed. Speed of chewing. Speed of swallowing. Speed of digestion. Speed of absorption. The person feels fed for a moment because the bloodstream has been supplied. The tissues are still asking a different question. Did enough structural material arrive to justify shutting appetite down.

That question matters because satiety is not just about calories entering the system. It is about whether the body senses that the meal delivered enough meaningful nutrition to reduce the need to keep seeking food. Refined carbohydrate often underperforms here because it is heavy in fast substrate and light in completion signals. Protein-linked satiety is weak because the amino acid load is weak. Fat-linked slowing of digestion is often weak unless the food is built as a hyper-palatable starch-fat mixture, which creates its own problems. The stomach empties relatively quickly. Glucose enters circulation quickly. Insulin rises quickly to contain it. The body receives a short-range fuel answer, but not much of a repair answer. That is why so many refined carbohydrate meals create the strange pattern of feeling filling and unfinished at the same time. The stomach was occupied. The organism was not fully satisfied.

The hormonal sequence reflects the same problem. A refined carbohydrate meal pushes early glucose handling to the front of the line. Insulin becomes the main immediate response because the body has to control what just entered. But stronger satiety hormones such as cholecystokinin and peptide YY are often less impressively engaged when the meal is low in substantial protein and natural fat. The digestive event becomes short and front-loaded. The body gets a sharp signal that fuel has arrived now, but a weaker signal that nourishment has arrived in a durable way. When that fast fuel is used or stored, hunger can return quickly because the deeper biological reason to stop eating never fully developed. The meal was handled. It was not truly finished.

This is one reason refined carbohydrate foods are so effective at driving repeated intake. They can be eaten easily, absorbed quickly, and rewarded strongly without resolving the body's broader structural and regulatory needs. Cereals, breads, pastries, crackers, snack foods, sweetened products, and many other refined carbohydrate staples can move a substantial calorie load into the body while supplying little complete protein, little useful fat, and weak micronutrient density unless those nutrients are added back artificially. Even then, fortification does not change the basic rhythm of the meal. It is still a fast glucose event built on a structurally thin foundation. The body gets energy. The body keeps looking for nourishment.

That is what it means to say refined carbohydrates often fail to finish the meal biologically. They do not merely digest quickly. They end the meal too early at the level of real satiety. They answer the urgent fuel question and leave the tissue question open. The person then experiences renewed hunger, cravings, or the pull toward more food not because appetite is irrational, but because the previous meal closed only part of the loop.

Why Persistent Hunger Is Often Biochemical, Not Moral

Persistent hunger is often interpreted as a character defect because modern nutrition keeps reducing appetite to choice. The person is told he lacks discipline, eats for comfort, gives in too easily, thinks about food too much, or fails to manage portions like a responsible adult. But the body does not generate hunger to make a moral point. It generates hunger when fuel access is unstable, when satiety signaling is weak, when structural nutrition is incomplete, or when the last meal failed to deliver enough usable material to convince the organism that real nourishment arrived. That is a biochemical event. A person can eat plenty and still remain hungry if the food was fast, low in complete protein, weak in useful fat, poor in micronutrient density, or engineered to stimulate reward harder than it stimulates completion. The appetite system then keeps asking because the biological problem is still open.

The chemistry of the meal explains much of this. A refined carbohydrate meal can raise blood glucose quickly, provoke insulin quickly, and create a brief sense of relief because immediate fuel entered circulation. But if that same meal is weak in protein and thin in natural fat, it often does little to slow gastric emptying, little to drive strong cholecystokinin and peptide YY signaling, and little to satisfy the body's structural demand for amino acids. The result is a meal that solved the fastest part of hunger and left the deeper part untouched. Blood sugar was handled. Tissue demand was not. The person then feels hungry again and is told he should have stronger willpower. The physiology is easier to read. The meal finished poorly. The body is still asking for completion.

Protein deficiency inside otherwise adequate calorie intake is one of the clearest versions of this problem. The body does not keep a large reserve pool of free amino acids, and it cannot build enzymes, immune molecules, connective tissue, gut lining, transport proteins, and muscle from carbohydrate alone. If meals repeatedly underdeliver complete, digestible protein, appetite can stay elevated because the organism is still trying to obtain substrate for repair. The same is true when fat is chronically underfed. Fat slows digestion, supports satiety, stabilizes post-meal energy, and changes how long the body can go without feeling metabolically urgent. When fat is stripped away and replaced with rapid carbohydrate, eating often becomes more frequent not because the person became weaker, but because the fuel pattern became shorter and more unstable.

Micronutrients shape hunger in quieter ways, but they still matter. A person can be overfed in calories and underfed in magnesium, zinc, iron, B vitamins, and other cofactors required for mitochondrial energy production, neurotransmitter balance, thyroid signaling, and general metabolic stability. In that state the body keeps receiving energy without converting it into stable function efficiently. Fatigue rises. Mood becomes more dependent on quick food relief. Cravings become easier to trigger. Appetite can then look emotional when part of the problem is still biochemical. The organism is trying to solve a deficit with the only lever it has, ask for more intake. That does not guarantee the next meal will solve the problem, especially if the next meal is built from the same low-yield processed inputs, but it explains why persistent hunger often feels stubborn and irrational. The body is searching through a poor food environment for something the previous food failed to supply.

This is why moral language makes the problem worse. Guilt does not improve bile flow. Shame does not raise protein quality. Self-criticism does not strengthen satiety hormones or improve amino acid delivery. If hunger is being driven by weak meal structure, unstable glucose handling, poor fat digestion, inadequate protein, or low nutrient density, then the solution is not more judgment layered on top of the same broken input. The solution is to feed the organism in a way that reduces the biological reason for hunger to stay active. Persistent hunger is often not a failure of virtue. It is the downstream behavior of a body that has been energized without being properly fed.

Chapter 25

Processed Food and Appetite Dysregulation

Hyper-palatable food changes appetite because it is designed to hit the reward system harder than the body's ordinary stopping signals can respond. This is not the same as food tasting good. A steak can taste good. Ripe fruit can taste good. Fresh butter can taste good. Hyper-palatability begins when softness, sweetness, saltiness, fat, flavor chemistry, and rapid mouthfeel are assembled in a way that makes continued intake unusually easy and unusually rewarding. The food dissolves quickly, requires little chewing, floods the mouth with sensory intensity, and keeps that intensity high across repeated bites. Real food usually carries some braking force. It asks for chewing. It asks for digestion. It generates satiety as amino acids and fatty acids begin entering the system. Hyper-palatable processed food weakens those brakes. Reward rises fast. Completion lags behind. The eater keeps receiving reasons to continue before the organism has had enough time to decide whether the meal actually solved anything.

This matters because appetite is partly governed by the relationship between sensory reward and nutritional resolution. In a coherent meal, those two things tend to move together. The food tastes good, digestion proceeds, satiety hormones rise, and the meal finishes biologically as the reward event is winding down. In a hyper-palatable processed meal, the relationship separates. Sweetness, salt, flavor enhancers, industrial fats, and soft refined starch create a powerful oral reward signal, but the structural value of the meal is often weak relative to that reward. Protein may be low. Micronutrient density may be thin. The digestive sequence may be too fast to build durable satiety before large amounts have already been eaten. The brain receives a strong message that this food is worth pursuing. The body receives a weaker message that it has been properly fed. That gap is where reward-driven eating lives.

The speed of intake makes the problem worse. Many processed foods are built to reduce friction at every step. Crunch collapses quickly. Creaminess requires almost no chewing. Refined starch and sugar move rapidly toward absorption. The person can consume a large energy load before cholecystokinin, peptide YY, gastric slowing, and the other deeper satiety signals have time to build. This is why processed snack foods, desserts, fast food combinations, sweetened cereals, and packaged convenience foods can feel almost unfinished while they are being eaten. The mouth keeps being impressed. The stomach and intestine are still trying to catch up. By the time they do, the energy load is already high and the person is left wondering why he kept going. The answer is not always weak character. Often the food was engineered to keep reward elevated while the biological stop signal remained delayed.

Reward-driven eating is therefore not just about pleasure. It is about nutritional mismatch. The food keeps stimulating pursuit after it stops making metabolic sense. It solves the immediate desire for taste and fast fuel while failing to close the deeper loop of satiety. The body may still be looking for amino acids, useful fats, and stronger nutrient density. Blood glucose may be rising and falling in a pattern that encourages more intake. The person may feel compelled to continue even though the meal is already calorically substantial because the calories arrived as reward more effectively than they arrived as nourishment. This is what processed food does so well. It teaches appetite to keep responding to intensity rather than to completion. Over time, that shifts eating away from biological regulation and toward repeated reward pursuit, which is exactly the environment in which appetite becomes hardest to trust.

Refined Food and Incomplete Nutrient Signaling

Refined food creates incomplete nutrient signaling because it delivers energy in forms the body can absorb quickly without delivering the full biochemical message that a substantial meal has actually arrived. The digestive tract is not only measuring calories. It is reading amino acid density, fat content, meal texture, gastric emptying speed, micronutrient load, and the hormonal sequence triggered as nutrients move from stomach to intestine to blood. A refined food built from flour, sugar, extracted oils, flavor systems, and synthetic fortification can send a very loud signal of reward while sending a much weaker signal of nourishment. Glucose appears quickly. Taste intensity is high. Insulin rises. The person feels fed for a moment. But protein-linked satiety may be weak, fat-mediated slowing may be thin or distorted, and the broader micronutrient context may be too poor to tell the organism that the meal solved anything beyond immediate fuel need. The body hears excitement. It does not hear completion.

This is why refinement changes appetite so powerfully. Whole or less-processed foods usually arrive with more resistance built into them. More chewing. More structure. More intact protein. More coherent fat. More time for the stomach and intestine to build a layered hormonal response. Refined foods strip much of that away. The meal moves faster. The bloodstream gets an earlier substrate hit. But the deeper signals that normally accompany real nutritional sufficiency are weakened because the food is thin where it counts. If complete protein is low, the body still lacks a strong amino acid message that repair material has arrived. If natural fat is weak or displaced by industrial mixtures, gastric slowing and bile-mediated digestion may not create the same satiety sequence. If micronutrient density is poor, the body may still be left with unresolved regulatory demand even while energy intake was high. This is incomplete nutrient signaling in practice. The meal says fuel is here now. It does not say the organism has been properly fed.

Fortification often hides this rather than fixing it. Adding vitamins and minerals back into a refined product can improve the label, but it does not necessarily restore the physiological meaning of the meal. The body is still receiving those compounds inside a food matrix built for speed, shelf life, and reward rather than for coherent digestion and satiety. A sweetened fortified cereal may carry added B vitamins and iron, yet still function mainly as rapid starch with weak protein density and poor completion. A "high protein" processed bar may advertise grams while delivering a compromised amino acid signal inside a matrix of sweeteners, syrups, flavor systems, and soft texture that encourages easy overconsumption. The label becomes more sophisticated. The nutrient signal can remain incomplete because the meal still does not behave like substantial nourishment.

This is why refined food keeps appetite active so effectively. It answers the fastest part of hunger and leaves the rest unresolved. The body receives energy, but not enough of the slower, denser information that tells it it can safely stop asking. Satiety hormones may rise, but not with the same force or duration. Blood glucose may be handled, but structural demand may remain open. The person then experiences this as a desire for more food, more flavor, more snacks, more constant intake. That is not always gluttony or weak self-command. Often it is the downstream effect of meals that stimulate reward harder than they communicate sufficiency. Refined food keeps the body metabolically half-convinced, and half-convinced bodies keep eating.

Why Industrial Foods Keep the Body Searching

Industrial foods keep the body searching because they are built to solve the easiest part of feeding while leaving the deeper biological job unfinished. They deliver energy rapidly, reward strongly, chew easily, and repeat well, but they often fail to deliver enough complete protein, enough useful fat, enough coherent micronutrient density, and enough slow digestive signaling to tell the organism that real nourishment has arrived. The mouth gets intensity. The bloodstream gets substrate. The tissues get a weaker message. That is the basic mismatch. A body that has been energized without being fully fed does not relax. It keeps looking.

This searching begins in the gut and continues in the endocrine system. Industrial foods are often soft, refined, sweetened, salted, and engineered to move quickly from hand to mouth to circulation. Refined starch breaks down fast. Sugar needs little preparation. Extracted fats raise energy density without necessarily creating the same biological completion that comes from a meal built around substantial protein and natural fat. The stomach may fill briefly, but gastric emptying, satiety hormone release, and amino acid signaling often fail to build the same durable stop signal. Cholecystokinin, peptide YY, and the broader satiety sequence respond more strongly when digestion is handling meaningful protein and fat, not merely a rush of processed substrate. So the person eats a lot, feels fed for a moment, and then feels the search reopen because the meal resolved urgency more than it resolved need.

Protein is central to this problem because the body keeps asking for structural material until it gets enough of it. Industrial foods are often poor at delivering dense, digestible, complete protein relative to their calorie load. That means a person can consume large amounts of processed food and still fail to satisfy the body's need for amino acids required for enzymes, immune proteins, gut lining turnover, connective tissue, and muscle maintenance. The same problem appears with micronutrients. A food may be fortified, but fortification does not automatically restore the full biological meaning of a coherent meal. The body may still be left low on the broader nutrient density that supports energy production, satiety, and metabolic steadiness. In that state appetite does not shut down cleanly because the organism is still waiting for the meal to become real.

Reward deepens the trap. Industrial foods stimulate wanting more effectively than they resolve needing less. They are designed to keep flavor high, texture easy, and sensory reward repeatable across many bites. That means the drive to continue can remain elevated even as the body falls short of nutritional completion. The eater experiences this as craving, snacking, grazing, or the strange urge to keep eating after a meal that was already calorically substantial. But the body is not confused. It is responding to a food environment that keeps delivering disposable energy and incomplete nourishment in the same package. The organism keeps searching because the meal kept promising more than it delivered.

This is why industrial foods can feel so hard to leave alone. They do not simply feed. They provoke. They create a body that is repeatedly stimulated, partly satisfied, and never fully convinced. Hunger in that environment becomes chronic not because the person is morally weak, but because the food keeps reopening the loop. Real nourishment tends to close it. Industrial food tends to keep it running.

Why Overeating Is Often Engineered Upstream

Overeating is often engineered upstream because the decision to eat too much is usually prepared before the eater feels out of control. It begins in the design of the food, the structure of the meal, and the metabolic state the previous meals have already created. A person does not typically arrive at overeating as a clean act of appetite failure in an otherwise neutral environment. He arrives there after repeated exposure to foods that are soft, refined, energy-dense, rapidly rewarding, weak in protein, often weak in micronutrient density, and poor at generating durable satiety. The body is then placed inside a sequence that keeps resolving the fastest part of hunger while leaving deeper nutritional demand partly open. The meal is incomplete before the second serving is taken. The overeating event is being set up earlier in the chain.

Food engineering is the first layer of that setup. Refined starch, sugar, industrial fat, salt, flavor chemistry, and low-friction texture create products that can be consumed quickly and rewarded intensely before the intestine has time to build a strong braking response. The eater gets sweetness, crunch, softness, creaminess, and rapid mouth reward all at once. Glucose enters circulation quickly. Insulin rises quickly. The stomach may contain a substantial calorie load, but the satiety pattern is weak relative to the energy delivered because complete protein is often low, natural fat context is poor, and the meal moved too fast to create durable completion. The person then keeps eating, not because the body is broken, but because the food was built to make continued intake easy while the deeper biological stop signal stayed delayed.

The second layer is metabolic priming. A person repeatedly eating glucose-heavy, low-structure foods often lives in a more unstable fuel environment before the next overeating event even begins. Hunger returns sooner. Blood sugar feels more volatile. Fat oxidation between meals is less available or less trusted. The body becomes more dependent on frequent external fuel because prior meals kept reinforcing short-range glucose handling rather than steadier substrate use. By the time the next meal begins, the organism is already more vulnerable to speed, reward, and repeated intake. In that state, overeating is not being created at the table alone. It was built by the earlier pattern of feeding that made the body easier to destabilize.

The third layer is environmental design. Portion sizes, convenience packaging, ready-to-eat formats, constant shelf availability, aggressive marketing, and the visual language of permission all remove barriers that once slowed intake naturally. A person is surrounded by foods that require little chewing, little preparation, little cost of decision, and little delay between impulse and consumption. That matters because friction is part of appetite regulation. When food must be prepared, chewed, and digested slowly, the body has more time to signal back. When food is engineered for immediate access and immediate pleasure, intake can outrun physiology. The person then appears to be making one bad choice, but the conditions that made that choice likely were installed long before he reached for the food.

This is why overeating is often engineered upstream. The excess intake at the end is real, but it is usually the final visible expression of food design, meal structure, hormonal timing, and environmental manipulation that were already working together. The body is not being asked a neutral question and then failing to answer it responsibly. It is being handed food that stimulates pursuit harder than it stimulates completion, inside a metabolic state shaped by previous meals that already weakened satiety and fuel stability. The overeating happens in the mouth and hand, but the machinery that made it likely was built much earlier.

Chapter 26

Insulin, Leptin, and Energy Partitioning

Insulin is not a moral hormone and it is not simply the molecule that makes carbohydrates controversial. It is one of the body's main distribution signals. Its job is to tell tissues that incoming fuel has arrived and that this fuel now needs to be moved, stored, or used according to immediate metabolic conditions. When glucose rises in the bloodstream after carbohydrate digestion, pancreatic beta cells release insulin. That release is not an abstract event. It changes what cells do. Muscle increases glucose uptake. The liver shifts toward glycogen production when capacity remains. Adipose tissue is pushed toward storage and away from release. Lipolysis, the liberation of stored fat, falls because the body is being informed that external fuel is already present. In other words, insulin changes traffic. It does not merely lower blood sugar in some isolated laboratory sense. It tells the organism how to handle the arrival of incoming energy.

This is why insulin has to be understood as both a storage signal and a distribution signal at the same time. Storage is the part people usually fixate on because it is easy to fear. But distribution comes first. The body cannot leave large amounts of glucose loose in circulation. Blood glucose must be controlled tightly, so insulin directs that glucose into tissues that can use it now or into storage sites that can hold it for later. Some goes into muscle as glycogen, the storage form of glucose. Some goes into the liver. Some contributes indirectly to fat storage when glycogen needs are met and energy keeps coming in. That outcome is real, but it is not proof that insulin is a villain. It is proof that insulin is a traffic director operating inside a body that has to manage incoming fuel intelligently or die from metabolic chaos.

The problem begins when insulin is forced to perform this role too often and under the worst dietary conditions. A meal built around refined starch and sugar sends glucose into circulation quickly. Insulin has to rise quickly in response. If this pattern happens again and again across the day, then the body spends more time in a fed-state storage posture and less time in a release posture. Stored fat becomes harder to access between meals because the signal to mobilize it keeps being interrupted by new glucose entry and new insulin release. The organism is therefore not only storing more easily. It is also being trained to depend more heavily on frequent incoming fuel. Appetite becomes more unstable because fast carbohydrate can solve the short-term energy problem quickly while leaving structural satiety incomplete if protein and fat are weak. The body is then living inside repeated distribution commands with too little metabolic quiet between them.

Insulin also changes what other nutrients mean once they arrive. Amino acids can stimulate insulin to a degree, but in the context of a protein-rich meal the broader message is different because amino acids are also signaling structural supply and are often accompanied by stronger satiety. Fat tends to blunt the speed of gastric emptying and changes the pace at which nutrients appear in circulation. Refined carbohydrate is different because it pushes the body most aggressively into immediate containment. That is why insulin cannot be discussed honestly outside food context. The same hormone is responding to very different meal structures, and those structures determine whether insulin is part of a coherent fed state or part of a repeated cycle of rapid fuel delivery and unstable appetite.

So insulin as a storage and distribution signal should be understood in sequence. Food enters. Glucose rises if carbohydrate was present in meaningful amount. Insulin rises in response. Tissues take up fuel. Glycogen is replenished where possible. Fat release is suppressed for the moment because external energy is already being handled. If that signal is occasional and metabolically appropriate, it is ordinary physiology. If it becomes the dominant rhythm of feeding through repeated refined carbohydrate exposure, it begins shaping the whole metabolic environment toward storage pressure, weaker access to stored fat, and more dependence on the next meal. Insulin is not the enemy in this story. It is the messenger revealing what kind of fuel pattern the diet keeps creating.

Leptin as a Long-Term Energy Status Signal

Leptin is the body's longer-range report on stored energy. While insulin responds quickly to the fuel arriving from the current meal, leptin reflects a broader condition. It is produced mainly by adipose tissue, and the amount released into circulation rises roughly in relation to how much stored fat the body is carrying. This makes leptin less like an acute feeding signal and more like a status update. The body is being told whether energy reserves are relatively abundant or relatively scarce. That signal reaches the brain, especially the hypothalamus, where appetite, energy expenditure, reproductive signaling, and broader survival priorities are being continuously adjusted. In simple terms, leptin helps tell the organism whether it is living in a state of reserve or a state of threat.

This matters because appetite is not governed only by what entered the stomach in the last few hours. It is also governed by what the body believes its longer-term fuel security looks like. When leptin signaling is working well, sufficient stored energy tends to suppress some of the urgency to keep eating and supports a more stable metabolic posture. The body is less defensive because reserves exist. When leptin falls, as it does with loss of body fat, prolonged calorie restriction, or other states of perceived energy scarcity, the organism becomes more protective. Hunger tends to rise. Energy expenditure may fall. Reproductive and thyroid-related functions may be downshifted. The body is not being dramatic. It is responding to what it interprets as a narrowing margin of safety.

The problem in modern metabolism is not usually the absence of leptin. It is that leptin's message becomes harder for the brain to interpret accurately. A person with substantial body fat often has substantial circulating leptin as well, yet appetite may remain high and energy regulation may remain unstable. This is commonly described as leptin resistance, though the phrase should be handled carefully because it can sound more final than the biology really is. The important point is that the signal is present, but the system is no longer responding to it cleanly. The brain is being told that stored energy exists, yet other aspects of the metabolic environment, repeated insulin exposure, chronic overfeeding of processed food, inflammation, poor sleep, stress signaling, unstable glucose handling, can distort how that message is received. The result is a body carrying energy reserves while still behaving partly as though it cannot trust them.

This is why leptin has to be understood as a long-term energy status signal rather than a simple appetite hormone. It does more than influence hunger in the next moment. It helps set the background metabolic attitude of the organism. Are reserves safe enough that intake can quiet down and energy can be spent more freely. Or does the body need to defend, conserve, and keep searching. When leptin signaling is distorted, appetite becomes harder to regulate because the body no longer reads its own energy stores clearly. A person can then feel both overfed and metabolically insecure at the same time, which is one of the defining contradictions of the modern food environment.

This is also why processed food and repeated glucose-heavy feeding can matter so much here. They do not just add calories. They help create the hormonal and inflammatory background in which long-term energy signaling becomes less trustworthy. Leptin is supposed to tell the truth about stored fuel. Modern metabolism often surrounds that truth with noise.

What Happens When These Systems Are Chronically Pushed

When insulin and leptin signaling are chronically pushed, the body does not stay in a simple fed state. It begins living in a distorted one. Repeated glucose-heavy meals, frequent snacking, hyper-palatable processed foods, poor sleep, and constant energy surplus keep insulin active too often and keep adipose tissue expanding under a hormonal climate that favors storage over release. At the same time, leptin rises with growing fat mass, but the brain stops responding to that signal with the same clarity. The result is a body carrying more stored energy while behaving less and less as if that stored energy is truly available and trustworthy. Hunger becomes harder to quiet. Fatigue becomes easier to trigger. The person can be overnourished in calories and underregulated in metabolism at the same time.

Insulin being pushed repeatedly changes fuel access first. If blood glucose is entering the system again and again, insulin keeps telling tissues that incoming fuel should be handled now and that stored fat does not need to be liberated. Lipolysis stays suppressed more often, which means the person becomes less practiced at moving cleanly between meals on internal fuel. Energy starts to depend more on the next intake and less on flexible access to reserves. This is one reason people can feel shaky, irritable, foggy, or compulsively hungry only a few hours after eating. The body is not just asking for food out of habit. It is living in a fuel environment that keeps pushing external energy through the front door while muting access to what is already stored in the basement.

Leptin being pushed chronically creates a different kind of distortion. In principle, rising fat mass should tell the brain that long-term energy reserves are abundant and that appetite can ease. But under chronic overfeeding, inflammation, sleep disruption, and repeated processed-food exposure, that message often loses force. The signal is high, but the interpretation is poor. The brain becomes less willing to trust that reserves are sufficient, so appetite remains more active than it should and energy expenditure may not rise in a way that fully compensates. This is how the body can become trapped in a paradoxical state. Stored energy is abundant. The regulatory system behaves as though security is still in question. The person keeps eating not because the body lacks fuel in absolute terms, but because the signaling systems that should calm intake and improve access to reserves have become noisy and unreliable.

The pancreas, liver, and adipose tissue all absorb this pressure over time. The pancreas is asked to produce insulin repeatedly. The liver is asked to manage continual glucose traffic, glycogen turnover, and in many cases rising substrate pressure from fructose and excess energy. Adipose tissue is asked not only to store more, but to function as a signaling organ under enlarging load. As adipose tissue expands, inflammatory signaling often rises with it, which further worsens insulin handling and disrupts leptin communication. The metabolic environment becomes more crowded and less precise. Glucose handling worsens. Appetite regulation worsens. Access to stored fat worsens. The body begins to feel less like a flexible fuel system and more like a machine that is always being fed and still somehow not fully satisfied.

This is where the lived experience becomes so confusing. A person may be carrying substantial body fat and still feel intense hunger. He may eat often and still feel low energy. He may consume large amounts of food and still experience cravings, crashes, and the sense that he is never fully done eating. That pattern is not well explained by morality. It is explained much better by a system in which insulin keeps pushing fuel into immediate handling and storage while leptin fails to communicate reserve sufficiency cleanly enough to quiet the drive for more intake. The body is being told two conflicting stories at once. Energy is abundant in storage. Energy does not feel reliably accessible. Appetite keeps trying to solve the contradiction.

When these systems are chronically pushed long enough, the result is not only weight gain. It is metabolic distrust. The body stops moving fluidly between fed and fasted states. It stops reading its own reserves calmly. Hunger becomes louder, satiety weaker, and fuel access more externally dependent. That is why repairing appetite usually requires more than eating less. The deeper task is to stop driving these systems into the same stressed pattern over and over so insulin can fall more appropriately between meals, leptin signaling can regain some credibility, and the body can begin trusting its own stored energy again.

Why the Modern Food Environment Keeps These Controls Unstable

The modern food environment keeps insulin, leptin, hunger, and satiety unstable because it keeps delivering the exact kind of input that these systems handle worst when repeated. It surrounds the body with foods that are easy to eat, fast to absorb, weak in structural completion, and available almost without interruption. Refined starch, sugar, industrial oils, sweet drinks, snack foods, desserts, packaged convenience meals, all of them push metabolism toward the same pattern. Glucose arrives quickly. Insulin rises quickly. Reward is high. Satiety is weak relative to the energy delivered. The person eats again before the previous meal has really resolved. The body then stops living in a rhythm of meal, absorption, use, and recovery. It begins living in a rhythm of constant re-exposure. That alone is enough to destabilize appetite regulation, because these control systems were not built for a day filled with repeated, low-friction, high-reward fuel events.

The instability is not only about food composition. It is also about food timing. The environment makes it normal to eat before the body has had time to shift meaningfully back toward stored fuel use. Breakfast cereal, coffee drinks, midmorning snacks, quick lunches, afternoon bars, sweetened beverages, dessert, evening snacking. Each one may look small in isolation. Together they keep insulin signaling active too often and keep the organism from spending enough time in the quieter space between meals where stored energy would normally become more available. Lipolysis stays interrupted. Glucose handling stays central. Hunger becomes tied more tightly to recent intake because the body is not being allowed to trust its own reserves. A metabolism repeatedly fed for speed becomes dependent on speed.

Processed food structure makes the same problem worse from the satiety side. Many modern foods are soft, rapidly consumed, easy to overeat, and weak in complete protein. They deliver energy without creating a strong enough stop signal. The stomach fills, but not for long. Blood glucose rises, but that is not the same as nutritional resolution. Cholecystokinin, peptide YY, and the other slower satiety signals do not get the same kind of decisive support they get from a meal built around substantial protein and natural fat. The brain receives intense reward. The tissues receive a weaker message that they have been properly fed. This is why the modern eater can be calorically saturated and still feel food-focused. The environment keeps provoking intake without closing the biological loop that would make intake settle down.

Sleep loss, stress, and constant sensory food exposure add another layer. A body sleeping poorly and living under chronic stress handles glucose less cleanly, reads hunger less calmly, and often seeks quicker reward because the broader regulatory environment is already unstable. Then the food environment meets that instability with exactly the wrong offer: fast fuel, high reward, low friction, everywhere. Even visual exposure matters. Food is no longer something encountered mainly at meals. It is present in gas stations, offices, apps, checkout lines, advertisements, and endless packaging cues. The appetite system is being stimulated before the digestive system is even involved. The body is being taught to anticipate food constantly, and anticipation itself changes behavior. A system repeatedly cued to expect reward becomes easier to push and harder to satisfy.

This is why the modern food environment does not merely tempt people. It trains the metabolism into instability. It keeps insulin active too often, keeps leptin signaling noisy, keeps satiety weak, keeps hunger reactive, and keeps stored energy less available than it should be between meals. The person then experiences this as poor self-control, constant cravings, or a metabolism that feels broken. But much of what looks like personal failure is really environmental design colliding with ordinary human physiology. The body is not malfunctioning in a vacuum. It is responding to a food environment built around repeated stimulation, repeated intake, and incomplete nutritional closure.

Part VIII

Building the Facultative Carnivore Diet

Chapter 27

Removing the Industrial Base of the Diet

Refined sugar is the cleanest example of why the modern diet became energetically rich and biologically thin at the same time. It enters the body as concentrated sweetness with almost no structural value attached to it. No meaningful protein. No meaningful fat. Very little of the mineral and vitamin context that would make it part of a serious feeding event. What remains is fast carbohydrate energy stripped of the physical resistance and nutritional depth that once limited how sugar behaved in the diet. The body can absorb it easily. That is the problem. A substance that arrives this quickly and this cleanly as sugar solves the shortest-range energy problem while doing almost nothing to solve the deeper problem of tissue nourishment. It lights up the mouth, enters the bloodstream, and changes insulin rapidly, but it does not tell the body that repair material has arrived, that membranes are being supported, or that a meal with durable satiety has just taken place.

The digestive sequence is almost insultingly short. Refined sugar does not ask much of the stomach. It does not require strong protein denaturation, meaningful bile-dependent fat handling, or prolonged enzymatic dismantling. It moves toward absorption with very little friction. Glucose can enter circulation quickly. Fructose, depending on the sugar source, is handled heavily by the liver, where it can contribute to glycogen repletion, lipogenesis, meaning new fat production, and a broader hepatic processing burden when exposure is frequent. This is why refined sugar changes metabolism so fast. It is not arriving as a complete food. It is arriving as a rapid substrate pulse. Insulin rises to contain the glucose fraction. The liver has to sort the fructose fraction. The eater experiences reward and quick energy. The organism experiences an abrupt fuel event that asks for management more than it offers nourishment.

That abruptness matters because appetite is not shut down by sweetness alone. A sweet food can feel satisfying in the mouth while remaining weak in the hormones and nutrient signals that actually finish a meal biologically. Refined sugar is poor at generating durable satiety because it carries almost none of the elements that make satiety strong. Protein is absent. Fat is absent unless added back in processed combinations that create other problems. Gastric emptying is not meaningfully slowed by the sugar itself. The result is predictable. The person gets quick relief, quick reward, and often a quick return of hunger or food-seeking because the body has not received the kind of meal that resolves structural demand. Sugar tells the system fuel is here now. It does not tell the system the organism has been properly fed.

This is why refined sugar becomes especially disruptive when it is no longer occasional and becomes part of the baseline architecture of the diet. A single sugary food is one metabolic event. Repeated daily sugar exposure is an endocrine climate. The pancreas is asked to handle repeated glucose entry. The liver is asked to process repeated fructose exposure and repeated excess substrate. Appetite learns to associate quick reward with incomplete completion. Energy becomes more volatile because the body keeps being pushed toward short-range glucose handling rather than calmer access to slower fuel. The person then feels pulled toward more frequent eating, more cravings, and more reward-seeking not because sugar is mysterious, but because it keeps reopening hunger after solving it only halfway.

So removing refined sugar is not mainly an act of purity. It is a structural correction. It removes one of the most efficient ways to flood the body with energy while starving the meal of real biological depth. Once refined sugar falls out of the foundation, appetite often becomes easier to read, energy less erratic, and meals more capable of finishing what they started. The goal is not to moralize sweetness. The goal is to stop building the diet around one of the fastest ways to feed the bloodstream and underfeed the body.

Refined Starch

Refined starch is what remains when a carbohydrate-rich plant food is stripped down until speed becomes its main virtue. Grain is milled, structure is reduced, fibrous barriers are weakened, and what reaches the eater is no longer a slow, defended plant tissue in any meaningful sense. It is a concentrated glucose source waiting for digestion to finish the job. The body does not receive refined starch as a complete food. It receives it as accelerated carbohydrate potential. Salivary and pancreatic amylase can break it down quickly. Brush-border enzymes finish the conversion into absorbable sugars. Glucose then enters circulation fast enough to create a strong insulin response even when the meal itself was nutritionally thin. That is the defining problem. Refined starch delivers a great deal of metabolic traffic while contributing relatively little to structural nourishment unless the rest of the meal compensates heavily.

This is why refined starch and whole carbohydrate-containing foods should not be discussed as though they are the same event with different branding. Intact plant structure creates friction. Fiber, water, cellular walls, tougher texture, slower chewing, and less efficient starch access all slow the rate at which glucose is liberated. Refinement removes much of that resistance. Bread, crackers, cereals, pastries, pasta made from highly milled flour, chips, snack products, and many processed staples all move in this direction. The digestive tract has less to dismantle and more to absorb quickly. The eater often experiences this as convenience or comfort. The body experiences it as rapid glucose entry with comparatively weak satiety and weak biological depth. A food can feel substantial because it is dense in starch. That does not mean it fed the organism well.

Refined starch is also poor at finishing appetite for the same reason refined sugar is poor at finishing it. It solves immediate fuel demand and leaves the deeper nutritional question unresolved. If a meal is built largely from refined starch and carries only modest protein and fat, the body receives fast glucose, insulin rises, glycogen may be replenished, and the person may feel briefly satisfied. But complete amino acids are still limited, useful fats may still be low, and the slower satiety signals built through meaningful protein digestion and bile-dependent fat handling may remain underpowered. The meal therefore resolves urgency more effectively than it resolves nourishment. Hunger can return sooner because the body did not get enough reason to stop asking.

The liver and pancreas absorb much of the cost here. The pancreas has to answer repeated starch-derived glucose entry with insulin. The liver has to sort, store, and redistribute that glucose load while keeping blood sugar within range between meals. When refined starch becomes a major dietary base, this is no longer an occasional fuel event. It becomes the dominant rhythm of feeding. The body is repeatedly pushed toward short-range carbohydrate management and away from quieter intervals where stored fat would normally become more relevant. Appetite becomes more reactive, energy more dependent on recent intake, and metabolic stability more vulnerable to the next gap between meals.

This is why removing refined starch matters in a facultative carnivore framework. The issue is not that all starch is evil in principle. The issue is that refined starch is one of the easiest ways to fill the diet with fast glucose while starving the meal of structural meaning. It teaches the body to live on rapid substrate turnover. It crowds out foods that provide complete protein, stable fat, and stronger micronutrient density. Once refined starch is removed from the base of the diet, meals stop behaving like short-term glucose events and start behaving more like actual feeding. That is the point. Not carbohydrate fear, but metabolic clarity.

Industrial Oils

Industrial oils are not just another source of fat. They are fats extracted, refined, and scaled for manufacturing in ways that separate them from the biological context in which fats were traditionally eaten. Soybean, corn, canola, cottonseed, sunflower, safflower, grapeseed, rice bran. These oils do not usually enter the food supply because people are pressing whole foods gently in the kitchen and consuming the result as a natural staple. They enter because modern processing can crush, solvent-extract, degum, refine, bleach, and deodorize them into shelf-stable ingredients that are easy to transport, easy to blend, and easy to pour into everything. That origin matters because it tells you what problem these oils were built to solve. They solve the industrial problem of cheap, scalable, neutral-tasting fat. That is not the same as solving the biological problem of how to nourish a body well.

The first issue is structural isolation. In a whole food, fat usually arrives inside tissue. It comes with protein, minerals, phospholipids, cholesterol, fat-soluble vitamins, connective structure, and a slower digestive context that makes the meal more coherent. Industrial oils strip the fat away from that broader architecture and deliver it as a concentrated extracted fraction. That changes the nutritional meaning of the fat immediately. The eater is no longer receiving a tissue. He is receiving an isolated energy input that can be added to starch, sugar, emulsifiers, flavor systems, and soft textures to create highly palatable food with weak structural value. This is why industrial oils are rarely a problem in isolation only. They usually appear inside foods already built around refined carbohydrate and low-friction intake. The oil raises energy density, extends shelf life, improves mouthfeel, and helps create repeatable overconsumption. The body gets more fuel. It does not necessarily get more nourishment.

The second issue is fatty acid profile and repeated incorporation. Many industrial seed oils are rich in linoleic acid, an omega-6 polyunsaturated fatty acid. Polyunsaturated fats are not inherently evil. The body uses them. But their chemistry matters. Double bonds make these fats more flexible and also more vulnerable to oxidation. When exposure becomes large and chronic, especially in a processed food environment already marked by excess energy, weak antioxidant support, and inflammatory stress, the body is being asked to incorporate more highly unsaturated fat into membranes and signaling pathways than it historically handled through intact foods alone. That matters because membrane composition changes signaling behavior, oxidative vulnerability, and the kinds of lipid-derived mediators the body produces. The issue is not that one serving of seed oil creates instant catastrophe. The issue is what kind of lipid environment repeated exposure helps build over time when these oils displace more stable animal fats and more coherent whole-food fat sources.

The third issue is thermal and manufacturing abuse. Industrial oils are often used in frying, repeated heating, shelf-stable packaged foods, and long storage conditions that expose them to heat, oxygen, and light. Unsaturated fats are more chemically fragile under those conditions. They can oxidize, fragment, and generate breakdown products that the body then has to absorb, detoxify, and manage. The liver inherits part of that burden. So does the membrane system once these altered lipids enter circulation. Again, the problem is not solved by saying the oil came from a seed and is therefore natural. Nature is not the relevant standard here. The relevant standard is what chemistry the oil arrived with, what chemistry storage and heating created, what digestion extracted, what the liver had to clear, and what kinds of fats were then incorporated into tissue.

This is why industrial oils belong with refined flour and sugar as part of the industrial base of the modern diet. They are cheap energy divorced from the tissue logic of real food. They make processed food richer without making it more complete. They help create meals that are calorie-dense, reward-heavy, and structurally weak. In a facultative carnivore framework, removing industrial oils is not mainly a purity ritual. It is a way of replacing extracted, chemically fragile, high-volume industrial fats with fats that arrive in more biologically coherent forms, butter, tallow, dairy fat, egg yolk, animal fat carried in meat, and other whole-food lipid sources that feed the body as part of an actual tissue package. The goal is not to fear fat. The goal is to stop outsourcing the fat supply to the cheapest oils the industrial system could mass produce.

Ultra-Processed Combinations

Ultra-processed combinations are where the industrial diet becomes most metabolically disruptive because the food is no longer just refined sugar, or refined starch, or industrial oil in isolation. It is all of them assembled into one continuous eating trigger. The starch is softened and made easy to digest. The sugar sharpens reward and accelerates intake. The extracted fat raises energy density and extends mouthfeel. Salt amplifies palatability. Flavor systems push the signal harder. Emulsifiers and stabilizers hold the product together in a texture that requires almost no effort to keep eating. This is not a meal that happened to become convenient. It is a product engineered so that reward rises faster than satiety, energy arrives faster than structure, and appetite stays active long after biological need should have started closing. The body is being given fuel in a form that outruns its own braking system.

The problem is not only that these foods are calorie-dense. It is that they deliver conflicting and incomplete signals at the same time. Refined carbohydrate pushes rapid glucose entry and a strong insulin response. Industrial fat slows gastric emptying enough to prolong the eating event and raise total energy load, but usually without the same satiety pattern that comes from a coherent meal built around substantial protein and natural fat. Protein is often weak, diluted, or heavily processed, so the amino acid signal for structural sufficiency remains underpowered. The mouth receives intensity. The bloodstream receives substrate. The tissues receive a thinner message that the meal actually supplied what the organism was looking for. This is why ultra-processed foods often feel both heavy and unfinished. They burden the gut and still fail to finish the meal biologically.

Texture makes the damage worse because texture changes timing. A pastry, a flavored chip, a sweetened cereal, a frozen dessert, a fast-food sandwich on a soft refined bun, all of them are built to reduce resistance. They chew quickly, dissolve quickly, and keep taste reward high across repeated bites. The person can consume a large amount of energy before the slower satiety systems, cholecystokinin, peptide YY, gastric slowing, and the broader hormonal sequence built around real digestion, have had time to answer. Intake runs ahead of physiology. That is why these foods are so easy to overeat. The person appears to lose control at the end, but the product was designed upstream so that control would be hardest exactly when the energy load became greatest.

Ultra-processed combinations also damage metabolic stability beyond the meal itself. Repeated exposure trains the body into a rhythm of fast fuel, repeated insulin signaling, weak satiety, and short intervals between eating episodes. Stored fat becomes less relevant because incoming glucose keeps arriving before the body has to lean on internal reserves. Leptin signaling becomes less trustworthy over time because the body is carrying more stored energy inside a food environment that keeps encouraging more intake anyway. Hunger becomes louder, cravings more frequent, and ordinary whole foods often start to feel less stimulating by comparison because the palate has been trained upward while the organism has been fed downward. The food keeps intensifying reward while thinning nourishment. That is the metabolic signature of ultra-processing.

This is why removing ultra-processed combinations matters more than arguing over individual ingredients in the abstract. The real damage is often in the stack. Fast starch plus sugar plus industrial oil plus low-friction texture plus artificial flavor coherence is a very different biological event from any one of those compounds alone. It creates a meal that overfeeds energy, underdelivers structure, weakens satiety, and teaches appetite to keep searching. In a facultative carnivore framework, clearing these foods out is not dietary theater. It is the removal of one of the most reliable ways to keep the body overexposed, underfinished, and metabolically noisy at the same time.

Why Removal Often Improves Stability Before Addition Does

The body often becomes more stable when the wrong inputs are removed before the right ones are added because physiology is easier to calm than to out-supplement. A system being hit all day with refined sugar, refined starch, industrial oils, and ultra-processed combinations is not merely undernourished. It is actively being pushed into volatility.

Glucose rises fast. Insulin rises fast. Appetite resolves poorly. The liver keeps sorting excess substrate. The gut keeps processing foods that are easy to absorb as energy and weak as nourishment. The person then tries to fix the problem by adding better foods, more protein, more liver, more eggs, more supplements, more minerals, more intention. But if the industrial base is still in place, the better input is being dropped into a system that is still being destabilized by the worse one. The body gets some benefit from the addition, but it is still spending much of the day managing noise.

This is why subtraction can have such disproportionate force. When refined sugar comes out, one of the fastest ways to create repeated glucose spikes and repeated incomplete satiety comes out with it. When refined starch comes out, the body stops being asked to solve so many short-range glucose events built on weak structural value. When industrial oils and ultra-processed combinations come out, energy density, reward intensity, and easy overconsumption often fall at the same time. The digestive tract has fewer chemically thin, reward-heavy meals to manage. The pancreas has fewer abrupt carbohydrate surges to contain. The liver has fewer repeated low-value substrate loads to sort and store. Appetite begins to quiet not because the person became morally better overnight, but because the metabolic environment became less chaotic. Removal works early because it reduces active interference.

Addition, by contrast, often has to fight through that interference if it is introduced too early. A person can add nutrient-dense animal foods, complete protein, natural fats, and even organ meats, but if those additions are laid on top of continued processed food intake, the appetite system may still be distorted, glucose handling may still be unstable, and the person may still keep eating in a way that buries the signal from the better food. The good meal becomes one event inside a day still dominated by engineered snacks, sweet drinks, refined starches, and unstable reward cycles. The body receives better material, yes, but it receives it inside a broader chemical climate that keeps reopening hunger and disrupting satiety. In that setting, better input is real, but removal would have done more to change the terrain.

There is also a simpler point. The body notices the absence of repeated insult faster than it notices the gradual arrival of deeper nourishment. Remove the constant glucose-heavy noise and blood sugar volatility may improve quickly. Remove the hyper-palatable processed stack and appetite often becomes easier to read quickly. Remove the industrial foods that keep the gut overexposed and digestive comfort may improve quickly. Those changes are not the full restoration of health, but they often create the first layer of stability that makes good additions finally land. Once the noise drops, protein works better as satiety. Natural fat works better as steady fuel. Organs and nutrient-dense animal foods begin filling real gaps instead of trying to compete with a constant stream of metabolic disruption.

That is why building a facultative carnivore diet usually works best in that order. First remove the foods that keep the body inflamed, over-signaled, underfinished, and metabolically rushed. Then add the foods that provide complete protein, usable fat, stronger micronutrient density, and better biological yield. Removal lowers the burden. Addition rebuilds the structure. If the burden is not lowered first, the rebuilding is slower and harder to feel.

Chapter 28

Rebuilding Around Protein and Fat

Establishing animal foods as the nutritional base means changing the order of nutritional judgment. The question stops being how to fit a little meat into a plant-centered diet and becomes how to build the diet on the foods that most directly meet human structural and regulatory needs. Animal foods move to the center because they deliver complete protein, usable fat, highly bioavailable minerals, and many critical vitamins in forms the digestive system can usually extract with high yield and relatively low friction. That is the practical meaning of base. Not exclusive in every case, not ideological, but foundational. These foods do the most work per unit of digestion. They give the body the raw materials it is repeatedly built from rather than forcing it to negotiate around fiber, antinutrients, weak amino acid profiles, and low-yield bulk as the main architecture of feeding.

This begins with protein because protein is the body's primary incoming structural substrate. Muscle, enzymes, transport proteins, immune molecules, connective tissue, gut lining turnover, repair after training, repair after ordinary life, all of it depends on amino acids arriving in sufficient quantity and in the right pattern. Animal foods tend to solve that problem cleanly. Meat, eggs, fish, and dairy do not merely contain protein. They provide complete essential amino acid profiles in forms digestion can denature, cleave, absorb, and route into the bloodstream with high efficiency. That immediately changes satiety, because meals built around real protein tend to finish the body's structural request more decisively. It also changes tissue maintenance, because the organism no longer has to work as hard to obtain what it was always built to need.

Fat matters just as much once animal foods become the base, because animal foods do not bring protein alone. They bring a lipid context that helps restore biological coherence to the meal. Natural animal fat slows digestion, supports bile-dependent handling, carries fat-soluble nutrients, contributes to membrane biology, and provides slower fuel that reduces dependence on repeated glucose delivery. This is important because a protein-centered diet without enough useful fat can become lean, hungry, and metabolically thin. The body does not only need amino acids. It also needs a stable fuel source, membrane material, cholesterol for steroid hormone production, and the digestive timing that fat helps create. When animal foods form the base, protein and fat arrive together in proportions that make the meal feel more like real feeding and less like a nutrient puzzle assembled after the fact.

Micronutrients widen the case further. Animal foods provide iron in a form the body absorbs more readily, vitamin B12 in a direct usable form, zinc without the same degree of binding interference found in many plant foods, retinol from liver and egg yolks, and a wide range of other compounds that arrive inside real tissue rather than inside fortification strategy. This is where the idea of biological yield becomes especially important. The body is not just getting numbers on paper. It is getting nutrients in forms that survive digestion and actually cross into circulation. Establishing animal foods as the base therefore changes the nutritional economy of the entire diet. Less total food volume is often required to obtain more usable nourishment. Appetite becomes easier to regulate because the meal delivers stronger completion. Digestion often becomes cleaner because the base of the diet is no longer built around defended plant structures and industrial combinations that require more negotiation.

This does not mean every non-animal food disappears automatically. It means the hierarchy becomes clear. Animal foods provide the foundation. Other foods are judged according to what they add, what they displace, what they cost to digest, and whether they improve or distort the system built on that foundation. Once that order is restored, eating becomes easier to think about. The body is fed first with the foods that most directly support structure, satiety, and stable energy. Everything else becomes optional, contextual, and secondary. That is what it means to rebuild around protein and fat. The diet stops orbiting cheap fuel and starts orbiting real nourishment.

Protein Sufficiency First

Protein sufficiency has to come first because the body cannot negotiate its way around missing structural material. It can adapt to lower carbohydrate. It can shift between glucose and fat as fuels. It can draw on stored triglyceride for energy over long periods. It cannot create essential amino acids out of stored fat or dietary philosophy. If protein is underdelivered, the organism begins making harder decisions immediately. Muscle maintenance weakens. Enzyme turnover becomes more constrained. Immune proteins, gut lining renewal, connective tissue repair, hormone signaling, and countless daily rebuilding tasks all compete for the same limited amino acid pool. That is why protein belongs at the front of the diet. Not because it is fashionable, but because it is the incoming substrate from which the body keeps replacing itself.

This changes how a meal should be judged. The first question is not whether it is low-carb, whole-food, clean, ancestral, or satiating. The first question is whether it supplies enough digestible, complete protein to meet the body's recurring structural demand. A meal can look metabolically clever and still fail here. It can be built around healthy fats, good intentions, and removed processed food while still underdelivering amino acids if protein density is too low. In that case the person may feel cleaner, but not necessarily better built. Hunger may remain louder than expected. Recovery may remain weaker than expected. Lean mass may remain harder to gain or keep. The body reads through all of that to the same deeper issue. Did real substrate arrive or not.

Protein sufficiency also changes appetite in a way few other dietary shifts can. When meals contain enough complete protein, the body receives a stronger amino acid signal that repair material is present in meaningful quantity. Satiety tends to rise because the meal is solving more than the next hour of energy. It is addressing tissue demand. This is one reason so many people can eat large amounts of processed food and still feel unfinished. The energy may have been high, but the protein signal was weak. The body was fed calorically and left structurally unsatisfied. Putting protein first changes that sequence. The meal becomes harder to outrun because it closes more of the biological reasons for continued intake.

This is also why quality matters as much as quantity. Protein sufficiency is not just about hitting a number with whatever happens to contain nitrogen. The body needs essential amino acids in the right proportions and in forms digestion can actually liberate and absorb. Animal foods matter here because they provide complete protein with high digestibility and a stronger leucine signal, which helps support muscle protein synthesis and broader repair. A lower-quality protein source may force the person to eat more volume, more total calories, and more digestive burden just to approach the same usable amino acid yield. So protein sufficiency first does not simply mean more protein in the abstract. It means enough high-yield protein to make the meal structurally decisive.

In practical terms, rebuilding the diet around protein and fat starts by making sure every serious meal clears this threshold before anything else is added around it. Build the plate on meat, eggs, fish, dairy, or other substantial animal foods first. Let starch, fruit, or plant foods remain secondary if used at all. That order matters because once protein is secured, the rest of the diet becomes easier to regulate. Satiety improves. Energy steadies. Lean tissue has a better chance of being maintained. Appetite becomes less frantic because the body is no longer chasing repair material through foods that were never rich in it to begin with. Protein sufficiency first is not a slogan. It is the point where the diet stops merely feeding the bloodstream and starts feeding the body.

Restoring Natural Fats

Restoring natural fats means putting fat back into its proper biological role after a long period in which it was treated mainly as a threat, a luxury, or a number to be minimized. The body never agreed with that downgrade. It kept building bile acids from cholesterol, storing and releasing bile through the gallbladder, packaging dietary lipids into chylomicrons, incorporating fatty acids into membranes, synthesizing steroid hormones from cholesterol, and relying on adipose tissue as its long-range fuel reserve. The physiology never changed. What changed was the diet. Natural fats were stripped out of meals and replaced with refined starch, sugar, industrial oils, and fortified low-fat products that looked controlled on paper while destabilizing hunger, glucose handling, and nutrient absorption in practice. Restoring natural fats is therefore not an indulgence. It is a return to giving the digestive system and the cells the lipid material they were always built to use.

The first effect is digestive. A meal with real natural fat slows down in the right way. It stimulates cholecystokinin, supports gallbladder contraction, improves the conditions for absorbing vitamins A, D, E, and K, and lengthens the digestive timeline so the body is not forced to live on rapid glucose appearance alone. That matters because satiety depends heavily on timing. A lean, starch-heavy meal can move fast, raise blood sugar fast, and leave the body metabolically unfinished fast. A meal built around protein and natural fat usually creates a more coherent sequence. The stomach empties more slowly. Nutrients arrive over a longer window. Satiety signals have time to build. Energy becomes less urgent because fuel is being delivered in a steadier stream. The body stops having to solve the same short-range carbohydrate problem over and over.

The second effect is structural. Natural fats are part of what cell membranes are made from. They support the lipid environment in which receptors, transporters, ion channels, and signaling systems actually function. Cholesterol is part of that architecture as well, helping stabilize membranes and serving as the precursor for steroid hormones. When natural fats are chronically displaced, the body does not simply lose calories. It loses part of the material economy that supports membrane integrity, hormone production, nervous system structure, bile chemistry, and fat-soluble nutrient handling. This is why adding back butter, egg yolks, dairy fat, tallow, the fat carried in meat, and other traditional animal fats often changes more than appetite alone. The body is receiving slower fuel, but it is also receiving structural lipid material in a form that still belongs to real food.

The third effect is metabolic. Natural fats help move the body away from dependence on repeated glucose rescue. As fat intake rises inside a diet built on adequate protein and lower industrial carbohydrate exposure, the organism begins leaning more confidently on fatty acid oxidation between meals. That does not mean carbohydrate becomes impossible or that glucose becomes irrelevant. It means the body is no longer trapped in a rhythm where energy feels stable only when another starch or sugar hit is close by. Higher-fat eating often makes the space between meals quieter because stored fat becomes easier to access and post-meal energy no longer depends so heavily on rapid glucose turnover. The appetite system changes with that shift. Hunger becomes less frantic because the body is not being trained into repeated short-range fuel dependence.

Restoring natural fats therefore means more than adding richness back to food. It means rebuilding a meal structure in which protein supplies amino acids, natural fat supplies slower fuel and lipid context, bile-driven digestion can work as intended, and fat-soluble nutrients can once again arrive with the medium required to absorb them. The goal is not to pour fat indiscriminately onto a broken diet. The goal is to replace industrial fats and glucose-heavy base foods with fats that still come packaged inside or alongside real tissue and real nourishment. That is how fat stops acting like a processed calorie source and starts acting like what it actually is in human physiology: structure, fuel, and signal.

How to Think About Carbohydrate Exposure

Carbohydrate exposure should be judged by timing, form, dose, and what the carbohydrate is displacing, not by the fantasy that all carbohydrates belong to one nutritional category. The body does not encounter "carbs" in the abstract. It encounters glucose potential arriving at a certain speed, inside a certain food structure, with a certain hormonal consequence. A ripe piece of fruit, a boiled potato, white rice, orange juice, bread made from refined flour, candy, sweetened cereal, and a pastry built from starch, sugar, and industrial fat are not the same physiological event simply because they all contribute carbohydrate. The question is always what kind of glucose burden is being created, how fast it reaches circulation, what insulin response it demands, whether the meal contains enough protein and fat to slow and stabilize the event, and whether the carbohydrate is helping a useful pattern or keeping the person trapped in repeated short-range fuel dependence. Carbohydrate is therefore not best understood as good or bad. It is best understood as exposure.

The first principle is that speed matters. Refined carbohydrate is usually the worst exposure because most of the structural resistance has already been removed. Flour, sugars, juices, sweetened products, and soft starch-heavy processed foods move quickly through digestion and create a fast-entry glucose event that the pancreas must contain through insulin. That makes them poor foundations for a stable diet because they keep training the body toward urgent fuel handling. Less refined carbohydrates, especially those still embedded in intact structure or used in simpler forms such as roots, tubers, or modest fruit intake, behave differently because digestion has to do more work before glucose appears in full force. Even then, context matters. A carbohydrate eaten alone acts differently from a carbohydrate eaten inside a protein-and-fat meal. The same potato can behave as a relatively calm addition to a steak-and-eggs style meal or as part of a high-glucose, low-satiety pattern depending on the rest of the plate and the rest of the day.

The second principle is that frequency matters as much as quantity. A single carbohydrate exposure and a diet built on repeated carbohydrate exposures are not the same biological decision. The body can handle glucose. That is not the issue. The issue is what kind of metabolic environment repeated glucose-heavy feeding creates. If carbohydrate is showing up in every meal, every snack, every drink, and every gap between meals, then insulin remains more active, lipolysis is interrupted more often, and appetite becomes easier to destabilize because the body keeps being taught to expect another fast fuel event before it ever has to rely deeply on stored fat. This is why many people feel better not simply when carbohydrate grams fall, but when carbohydrate stops defining the rhythm of the entire day. A body that sees carbohydrate occasionally is one thing. A body that must keep seeing it to feel normal is another.

The third principle is that carbohydrate should be treated as secondary fuel, not as the structural center of the diet. Protein comes first because it supplies the amino acids the body cannot make and cannot store deeply. Natural fat comes next because it stabilizes digestion, supports membranes and hormones, and provides slower fuel. Once those are established, carbohydrate can be judged more honestly. Does it support training, recovery, body size, tolerance, sleep, or personal preference without destabilizing appetite and energy. Or is it crowding out the foods that actually build the organism while pushing the person back into glucose dependence. In a facultative carnivore framework, carbohydrate is not automatically banned and not automatically required. It is conditional. It earns its place by fitting the body rather than by inheriting the status of a default staple.

So the right way to think about carbohydrate exposure is not to ask whether carbohydrate exists in the diet, but how much of the diet's metabolic rhythm is being organized around it. If the person is hungry again too soon, needs frequent eating to stay functional, lives on quick glucose relief, or keeps displacing dense animal foods with starch and sugar, the carbohydrate burden is too high for that body in that context. If carbohydrate is limited to simpler forms, used in amounts the person handles well, and kept subordinate to protein and natural fat, it may be tolerated without dominating the system. The body can use carbohydrate. It simply should not be forced to live at its mercy.

How to Think About Plant Foods as Optional, Not Foundational

Plant foods become easier to judge once they are removed from the position of automatic dietary authority. The usual nutrition framework begins by treating fruits, vegetables, grains, legumes, nuts, and seeds as the unquestioned base of a healthy diet, with animal foods added around the edges as secondary support. A facultative carnivore framework reverses that hierarchy. Animal foods become foundational because they provide complete protein, useful fats, fat-soluble nutrients, highly bioavailable minerals, and strong satiety with relatively direct digestion. Plant foods then move into a different category. They are no longer protected by reputation. They are judged by contribution, cost, and compatibility. What do they add. What do they displace. What do they demand from digestion. What chemistry do they bring with them. What is the net biological result after the full interaction is over. Optional does not mean forbidden. It means no longer assumed necessary simply because nutrition culture assigned them that role.

That change matters because many plant foods are nutritionally mixed events. They may provide carbohydrate, flavor, texture, color, variety, or in some cases useful vitamin and mineral contribution. But they also arrive with fiber, antinutrients, defense compounds, incomplete protein, weaker mineral availability, fermentation burden, and a higher dependence on host tolerance and preparation. A root or fruit may be tolerated well in modest amounts by one person and destabilize appetite or digestion in another. A leafy green may look mineral-rich on paper while delivering much less once oxalate binding and gut chemistry become real. A nut may be praised for nutrients while also arriving as a package of phytate, fiber, and calorie density with limited protein efficiency. Once plant foods are treated as optional, the body no longer has to pretend these tradeoffs do not exist. The food can be judged honestly.

Thinking of plant foods as optional also protects the structural base of the diet. If the meal is built first around substantial animal protein and natural fat, then any plant food that is added is entering a system already anchored by real nourishment. That means the plant food can be judged for whether it improves the meal or merely dilutes it. A small amount of fruit, a serving of a well-tolerated root, or a modest vegetable side may be harmless or even useful in that context. But if plant foods dominate the plate, the risk rises that protein density falls, fat falls, satiety weakens, and digestion becomes more dependent on negotiating defended plant matter rather than absorbing dense animal nutrition. Optional means the plant food has to earn its place. It is not allowed to take the foundation for granted.

This also changes the emotional tone of the subject. Plant foods no longer need to be worshipped or feared. They can be treated as variables. Some people will tolerate more. Some will tolerate less. Some foods will work seasonally, contextually, or in modest quantity. Others will repeatedly create bloating, unstable appetite, bowel irritation, oxalate burden, or simple displacement of better food. Once the foundational status is removed, the person is free to ask the only question that matters. Does this food help this body under these conditions, or does it add friction. That is a more serious and more biologically honest question than whether the food belongs to a culturally approved category.

So to think about plant foods as optional, not foundational, is to stop treating them as the default architecture of nourishment. The default architecture becomes animal foods because they feed the organism more directly. Plant foods then become conditional additions whose value depends on tolerance, preparation, dose, and what they are replacing. Some may fit. Some may not. None need to be granted automatic nutritional authority before the body has even spoken.

Chapter 29

Practical Implementation

Meal structure matters because the body does not eat ingredients one at a time. It eats sequences. A meal enters the digestive tract as a combined physiological event, and the order of that event determines whether the body experiences the food as stabilizing or chaotic. If the plate begins with refined carbohydrate, weak protein, and little natural fat, digestion tends to move fast, glucose enters early, insulin rises early, and satiety often arrives late and weak. The body solves the short-range fuel problem before it has received enough reason to stop asking for food. A well-structured meal does the opposite. It begins with the nutrients that feed the organism most directly and that create the strongest completion signal once digestion begins. Protein first. Natural fat with it. Everything else arranged around that foundation rather than competing with it. That is not a slogan. It is a way of making the meal legible to the body.

In practical terms, this means every serious meal should be built on a substantial animal protein source and enough natural fat to make the meal digest more slowly and finish more completely. Meat, eggs, fish, dairy, or combinations of these should carry the center of the plate because they provide the amino acids and lipids that most directly support satiety, tissue maintenance, and metabolic steadiness. The meal should look anchored, not padded. A person should be able to identify immediately where the protein is, where the fat is, and whether the plate is built to feed the body or merely to occupy it. Once that foundation is in place, any carbohydrate or plant food that remains can be judged honestly. Is it small enough not to take over the meal. Is it simple enough not to create unnecessary digestive noise. Is it helping the meal or diluting it. This is what meal structure clarifies. It prevents side foods from becoming the real food.

The timing of eating matters too, but timing only makes sense after structure is corrected. A body fed on dense protein and natural fat often does not need to be managed constantly because those meals tend to digest more slowly, suppress hunger more effectively, and allow the person to move further between meals without strain. That means meal structure should favor real meals over grazing. A meal should be large enough and complete enough that the body has time to digest, absorb, and use it before the next feeding event begins. Constant snacking usually keeps insulin more active, interrupts access to stored fuel, and teaches appetite to expect external input before the last meal has even been metabolically resolved. A well-structured day therefore tends to have fewer, stronger meals rather than a continuous stream of small, weak ones.

This is also why meal structure should be judged by what happens afterward. The right meal leaves the person calm, fed, and less interested in food for a meaningful stretch of time. It does not create a quick rise followed by a pull toward more eating. It does not leave the stomach mechanically full and the body nutritionally unfinished. It does not rely on sweetness, crunch, novelty, or constant variety to stay appealing. It feeds the organism first. When meal structure is correct, appetite becomes easier to interpret because the body is no longer being asked to solve nourishment through guesswork. A meal should not merely fit macros on paper. It should create a coherent digestive event that ends with the organism more stable than it was before eating.

Satiety-Based Eating

Satiety-based eating begins with a different question from the one most people are taught to ask. The usual question is how little can I eat without losing control later. Satiety-based eating asks what kind of meal actually closes the loop. That shift matters because the body does not stop asking for food when enough discipline has been performed. It stops asking when the meal has delivered enough meaningful material, enough complete protein, enough useful fat, enough digestive timing, and enough hormonal confirmation that nourishment has truly arrived. A person can portion-control a weak meal and still remain biologically unfinished. He can also eat a larger meal built around dense protein and natural fat and find that appetite disappears because the organism no longer has reason to keep searching. Satiety-based eating therefore does not mean eating until physically stuffed. It means eating until the body has enough reason to quiet down.

That only works if the meal is structured correctly. Satiety cannot be trusted well when the plate is built on refined carbohydrate, sweetened drinks, snack foods, weak protein, and industrial combinations designed to keep reward high while completion stays low. In that setting, appetite signals become noisy because the food solved urgency more than nourishment. Satiety-based eating has to begin with real meals. Substantial animal protein. Natural fat. Enough food volume to create a genuine digestive event rather than a brief glucose episode. When meals are built this way, satiety becomes more readable because it is being generated by amino acid sufficiency, slower gastric emptying, bile-dependent digestion, and a stronger hormonal sequence involving cholecystokinin, peptide YY, and other signals that actually correspond to biological completion. The body is easier to trust when it is being fed honestly.

This also means satiety-based eating requires stopping the habit of interrupting appetite before it can reveal itself clearly. Constant snacking, grazing, sipping calories, and eating on schedule regardless of hunger all blur the signal. If the person is repeatedly giving the body small amounts of quick fuel, he never really sees what a complete meal would have done or how long it would have carried him. Satiety-based eating works best when meals are distinct and allowed to finish their job. Eat enough at the meal to create real completion, then allow the body to live off that meal rather than immediately layering another one on top. That spacing teaches the metabolism to trust slower fuel again and helps expose whether the meal was truly adequate. A meal that was real can carry time. A meal that was mainly quick glucose usually cannot.

The practical test is not how noble the meal looked or how perfectly it matched a spreadsheet. The practical test is what happened afterward. Did hunger stay quiet for a meaningful stretch without white-knuckling. Did energy remain reasonably stable. Did the person stop thinking about food because the body was fed, or did the mind keep circling back because the meal was incomplete. Satiety-based eating pays attention to those downstream results. It treats them as information rather than as evidence of moral success or failure. If the person is hungry too soon, the answer is often not stricter control. It is usually that the previous meal was too small, too low in complete protein, too low in natural fat, too high in refined carbohydrate, or too weak in overall biological yield.

This is why satiety-based eating fits a facultative carnivore framework so well. Once the meal is anchored by substantial animal food and enough natural fat, appetite becomes less theatrical. The person does not need constant tricks, stimulants, sweeteners, or emotional management to get through the day. He eats, gets fed, and moves on. That is the goal. Not endless self-surveillance, but a meal pattern strong enough that the body stops arguing with it.

Food Selection by Biological Yield

Food selection by biological yield means judging food by what the body is actually left with after digestion, absorption, transport, tissue use, and clearance are over. That is a very different standard from choosing food by label, reputation, calories, or cultural status. A food can look impressive on paper and still yield very little if its protein is incomplete, its minerals are bound, its fats are poorly handled, or its carbohydrate load destabilizes appetite without supplying much structural value. Another food can look plain, even unfashionable, and still outperform it because digestion can liberate dense amino acids, usable fats, fat-soluble nutrients, and bioavailable minerals with relatively little friction. Biological yield asks the harder question. Not what does this food contain in isolation, but what can the organism actually extract, retain, and use after the full event is over.

That standard changes food choice immediately. A steak, eggs, full-fat dairy, fish, and other substantial animal foods tend to rank highly because they deliver complete protein, useful fat, strong satiety, and micronutrients in forms the human digestive tract handles directly. The stomach can denature the protein, pancreatic proteases can reduce it into amino acids, bile can emulsify the fat, the intestine can absorb the resulting nutrients with high yield, and the tissues can use much of what arrives without extraordinary conversion or cleanup cost. By contrast, many foods that carry a health reputation lose force under this standard. A fortified cereal may contain added vitamins and minerals, but the real event is still refined starch moving rapidly into circulation with weak protein value and incomplete satiety. A leafy plant may test high in calcium, yet oxalate can bind much of that calcium before absorption. A nut may carry minerals and fat, but also phytate, fiber, and lower protein efficiency. The number survives on the label. The body receives a smaller return.

Biological yield also forces food selection to include cost, not just content. Some foods nourish with relatively low digestive and metabolic friction. Others make the body work harder for a thinner result. The cost may show up in different places. More gastric effort for poor protein extraction. More bile demand for low-value processed fat. More fermentation burden in the colon from poorly digested plant material. More insulin traffic from refined carbohydrate. More renal handling of compounds the body cannot meaningfully use. Once this is taken seriously, the best foods are not simply the foods with the longest nutrient panel. They are the foods that produce the best ratio of usable nourishment to digestive burden. That is why food selection by biological yield tends to favor dense animal foods, natural fats, eggs, dairy when tolerated, and other foods that meet the body where its digestive architecture is strongest.

This way of choosing food also simplifies appetite. The body usually becomes less noisy when meals are built from foods with high biological yield because those foods tend to close more of the nutritional loop in one sitting. Complete protein lowers unresolved structural demand. Natural fat slows digestion and extends satiety. Better micronutrient density improves the chances that the energy in the meal can actually be converted into stable cellular work. Processed foods often do the opposite. They overdeliver energy while underdelivering completion, which keeps the body searching. High-yield foods reduce that search because they give the organism more of what it was asking for in the first place.

So food selection by biological yield is not a branding strategy or a purity game. It is a physiological filter. Choose the foods that digestion can turn into real nourishment with the least waste, the least interference, and the strongest structural return. Demote the foods that look impressive but leave the body underfed, overburdened, or metabolically unstable. That is how food choice stops being about reputation and starts being about what the organism actually gains.

Organ Rotation

Organ rotation works because organ meats are concentrated, not because they are magical. The mistake is to treat them either as exotic superfoods that must be eaten constantly or as strange relics that have no place in a modern diet. Both views miss the tissue logic. Liver, heart, kidney, marrow, spleen, and other organs do not function like ordinary muscle meat. They carry different nutrient densities because they performed different jobs inside the animal. Liver concentrates retinol, copper, folate, vitamin B12, riboflavin, and a broad range of regulatory compounds because it was a storage and processing organ. Heart reflects continuous oxidative work. Kidney reflects filtration and biochemical sorting. Marrow and connective tissues widen the fat and collagen economy of the diet. Rotation matters because no single organ represents the whole animal any more than muscle meat does. Different tissues widen nutrient coverage in different directions.

The practical value of rotation is that it lets the body receive this density repeatedly without forcing one organ into the role of daily staple. Liver is the clearest example. It is rich enough that a small amount changes the nutritional profile of the week, not just the meal. That means the goal is not to eat liver like ground beef. The goal is to use it periodically so retinol, copper, B12, folate, and related cofactors re-enter the diet in meaningful concentration. Heart can appear more often because it behaves more like a dense working muscle with a different micronutrient pattern. Marrow, skin, broth, and connective cuts can widen collagen-rich intake and natural fat intake without needing special ritual. Rotation keeps the diet broad at the tissue level while remaining practical at the table.

This also solves a modern problem of nutritional monotony. Many people technically eat animal food while still narrowing the diet to a small set of lean muscle cuts. That can produce strong protein intake, but it leaves part of whole-animal nutrition unused. Organ rotation restores some of that lost range without making every meal complicated. A little liver once or twice a week, heart worked into ordinary meat dishes, marrow or collagen-rich cuts used regularly, and occasional use of other organs as tolerated can shift the nutrient field substantially. The body then stops depending so heavily on supplements or fortified foods to imitate what tissue diversity once supplied naturally.

Rotation should therefore be guided by density, tolerance, and sustainability rather than by ideology. Use small repeated exposures. Let muscle meat remain the main structural base. Let organs deepen the regulatory side of the diet. The goal is not performance eating. The goal is to widen micronutrient coverage through real tissues in amounts the body can use and the person can maintain. That is what organ rotation does when it is understood correctly. It turns whole-animal nutrition from an abstract principle into an ordinary pattern of feeding.

Digestive Adaptation During Transition

Digestive adaptation during transition is not a vague detox phase or a mystical reset. It is the body adjusting to a new mechanical and chemical workload. A diet built around refined starch, sugar, industrial oils, snack foods, and frequent eating trains digestion toward speed, not depth. Meals move quickly. Glucose handling dominates. Bile-dependent fat digestion may be used less forcefully. Satiety is often built poorly and appetite stays noisy. When the diet shifts toward substantial animal protein, natural fat, fewer eating episodes, and less refined carbohydrate, the digestive tract has to change its rhythm. The stomach may need to hold food longer and acidify more strongly. The gallbladder may need to release bile more decisively. Pancreatic output may need to match a heavier protein-and-fat meal pattern. The intestine has to process a diet that is denser, slower, and more structurally meaningful. That shift is real physiology. It is not failure when the body notices the difference.

The first place this often shows up is in fat handling. A person coming from years of lower-fat eating or from a diet dominated by processed carbohydrate may feel heaviness, bloating, loose stool, pale stool, or a sense that richer meals just sit there. That does not automatically mean the higher-fat pattern is wrong. Often it means bile flow, gallbladder contraction, meal pacing, and digestive coordination have not yet caught up to the new demand. Fat requires emulsification, micelle formation, and lymphatic transport. If the liver, gallbladder, and pancreas have spent years working against a different dietary rhythm, the transition can expose weakness. The body is being asked to digest fat as real food again rather than to live mainly on rapid glucose traffic. Some adaptation is simply the digestive system relearning how to do that job consistently.

Protein can create its own transition issues for the same reason. Dense animal protein asks more of the stomach than processed food does. It needs acid, pepsin activation, churning, pancreatic proteases, and enough time for proper breakdown before the amino acids can be absorbed. A person who has lived on soft, fast, low-protein food may initially experience large protein meals as heavy, not because protein is the problem, but because the digestive sequence has been underused or poorly coordinated. Fast eating makes this worse. A high-protein meal swallowed quickly is much harder to process than the same meal eaten with enough chewing and enough time for the cephalic phase and gastric phase to organize themselves. During transition, meal construction and pace matter. Real food cannot be eaten like snack food without consequences.

The appetite system also adapts. People coming from a glucose-heavy pattern are often accustomed to frequent eating because their meals solved urgency more than nourishment. When protein and fat rise and meal frequency falls, the body has to relearn what full satiety and slower fuel delivery feel like. In the beginning, this can feel confusing. Hunger may come at familiar clock times even when the body is still metabolically supplied. Cravings may persist because reward circuits were trained around rapid carbohydrate and constant stimulus. That does not mean the new structure is failing. It often means the old structure is still echoing. Real satiety tends to become clearer only after the body has enough repeated exposure to meals that actually finish the meal biologically.

This is why transition should be approached as digestive retraining rather than as immediate proof of concept. Meals should be large enough to matter, but not so extreme that digestion is overwhelmed before adaptation begins. Protein should be substantial and regular. Natural fat should be restored steadily, not hidden from. Eating speed should slow down enough for digestive preparation to occur. Refined sugar, refined starch, industrial oils, and ultra-processed combinations should fall away early, because they keep the old metabolic rhythm alive and make adaptation harder to read. As that industrial noise drops, stomach acid often becomes more useful, bile signaling becomes more relevant, appetite becomes less frantic, and the body starts to trust slower fuel again. Digestive adaptation during transition is therefore not a side issue. It is part of how the body moves from living on quick substrate and incomplete satiety to living on denser meals that actually nourish.

Common Friction Points and How to Solve Them

Most friction points in a facultative carnivore transition are not signs that the framework is wrong. They are signs that the body is moving from one metabolic and digestive pattern into another and that some part of the old pattern is still exerting force. The common problems usually cluster around the same places. Appetite timing, fat digestion, meal size, protein sufficiency, bowel changes, salt and fluid balance, and the psychological pull of processed food reward. If these are misunderstood, the person starts negotiating against the diet too early. If they are read correctly, they become useful feedback. The question is not whether friction exists. The question is what kind of friction it is. A body that feels hungry too soon is often underfed in protein or still overexposed to refined carbohydrate. A body that feels heavy after higher-fat meals may be showing weak bile coordination, rushed eating, or too abrupt a jump in fat load. A body that feels flat, headachy, or irritable in the early phase may be shifting fuel systems while also losing sodium and water as insulin falls. These are different problems and they need different corrections. Lumping them all together as "adaptation" is too vague to help.

The first major friction point is weak satiety despite eating more animal food. In practice this usually means the meals are still too small, too lean, too snack-like, or too mixed with foods that keep glucose handling dominant. A person may say he is eating meat, but if the meal is built around a small portion of lean protein with fruit, starch, or low-fat side foods doing most of the caloric work, the body is still being trained into the old rhythm. The solution is usually straightforward. Increase the actual protein load. Build the meal around a real serving of meat, eggs, fish, or dairy that can create a decisive amino acid signal. Stop being timid with natural fat if the meal is too lean to satisfy. Remove the side foods that are reopening appetite before the protein-and-fat base can finish the meal biologically. Another common issue is eating too often. Frequent eating can blur whether the meal was truly adequate because the person never gives the body enough time to reveal its real satiety response. Stronger meals and fewer eating episodes usually solve more than tighter portion rules ever will.

The second friction point is digestive discomfort with richer meals. Heaviness, bloating, nausea, loose stool, greasy stool, upper abdominal pressure, or the sense that fat just sits there usually point toward bile and pacing rather than toward some abstract inability to eat animal food. The body may simply be underprepared for larger fat loads after years of lower-fat or highly processed eating. The solution is not to panic and run back to refined carbohydrate. It is to improve the mechanics. Slow the meal down. Chew properly. Do not make every meal a massive fat test. Use moderate but consistent natural fat instead of alternating between very low fat and very high fat meals. Give the gallbladder repeated real reasons to contract. If symptoms are strong and persistent, that suggests a more meaningful issue with bile flow, gallbladder function, pancreatic contribution, or broader digestive health, and the answer is to address that physiology directly rather than pretend the food itself was the error. The same logic applies to protein heaviness. Large meat meals eaten too fast or on a weak acid foundation often feel worse than the same meals eaten more slowly and more consistently.

The third friction point is low energy, headaches, irritability, cramping, or the sense of feeling strangely depleted during the first phase of carbohydrate reduction. Very often this is not a protein problem or a calorie problem first. It is an electrolyte and fluid problem. As insulin falls, the kidney tends to release more sodium and water. Glycogen also drops, and glycogen carries water with it. A person can therefore feel worse not because the body needs more cereal or sugar, but because the body is losing fluid and sodium while fuel handling is changing. The fix is practical, not mystical. Salt food more deliberately. Use broth if needed. Do not under-eat while also pulling carbohydrate down sharply. Keep protein strong and let natural fat rise enough that meals are not turning into lean, unsatisfying austerity. Many people interpret this temporary instability as proof that carbohydrate was biologically required at high levels. Often it is simply proof that the transition was under-salted and underfed.

The fourth friction point is bowel change. Some people become looser at first, especially when bile flow is still adapting or when the shift away from starch-heavy, fiber-heavy eating is abrupt. Others become more constipated because meal size is too small, sodium is too low, fluid intake is poor, or fat digestion is incomplete. This is where people often get trapped by old assumptions. They immediately conclude they need to add back large amounts of fiber because stool volume fell, when stool volume and bowel function are not the same thing. Less residue is expected when the diet contains more highly digestible animal food and less indigestible plant bulk. The real question is whether transit is comfortable and regular, not whether the bowel output looks impressively large. If constipation appears, first check food quantity, protein adequacy, salt, fluid, and fat handling before assuming the answer is more plant roughage. If bloating and excess gas remain high, that often means too much fermentable carbohydrate or too much unfinished material is still reaching the colon.

The final friction point is reward pull. Processed food cravings, emotional attachment to sweet foods, the urge to snack, and the feeling that meals are too plain usually reflect the fact that appetite is not only adapting to new nutrients. It is withdrawing from chronic overstimulation. A diet based on real animal foods will often feel quieter than a diet built on ultra-processed combinations, and quiet can feel like deprivation to a palate trained on constant intensity. The solution is not to chase novelty through packaged "carnivore" desserts or highly manipulated substitutes. That simply keeps the reward machinery alive in a different costume. The better solution is repetition, substantial meals, enough salt, enough fat, and enough actual satisfaction that the body stops feeling biochemically unfinished while the reward system slowly comes down from its old baseline. Most people do not need more tricks. They need enough exposure to real satiety that processed food stops feeling necessary.

So the common friction points are usually readable if the framework stays physiological. Too hungry usually means the meal was too weak, too lean, too small, or too interrupted. Digestive heaviness usually means the fat or protein load outran digestive coordination. Headaches and flat energy often mean sodium and fluid dropped while metabolism was shifting. Bowel changes often mean the person is misreading less residue as dysfunction or ignoring simple issues of food quantity and fat handling. Cravings often mean the reward system is louder than the satiety system, at least for a while. Solve the mechanism, not the mood around it. That is how friction becomes information instead of derailment.

Chapter 30

Flexibility, Context, and Sustainability

The word *facultative* matters because it protects the framework from becoming another dietary prison. It means the body has a center without being trapped in a single narrow expression of that center. A facultative carnivore framework does not argue that human physiology collapses the moment a plant food appears on the plate or that every person must eat the same foods in the same amounts under all conditions. It argues something more precise. Animal foods appear to provide the most direct route to structural nourishment, stable satiety, and efficient nutrient delivery, but the body still retains flexibility around that base. Flexibility is built into the term itself. The mistake is to hear flexibility and erase hierarchy, or to hear hierarchy and erase flexibility. *Facultative* keeps both. It says there is a nutritional center of gravity, and it also says the organism can move around that center without turning every deviation into a biological crisis.

That matters in real life because no serious dietary pattern survives long if it confuses precision with brittleness. Appetite changes. Training changes. Season changes. Illness changes demand. Social life changes what is practical. A person may tolerate certain fruits, roots, or fermented plant foods well in one period and prefer fewer of them in another. Another person may function best with a much tighter animal-food pattern because digestion, appetite, bowel function, or metabolic stability deteriorate once plant load rises. Both realities can exist inside the same framework because the framework is not built on ideological purity. It is built on biological fit. The question is not whether a food violates a rule. The question is whether the food helps or destabilizes the organism in that context. A rigid diet asks for loyalty. A facultative framework asks for honest observation.

This is also why the word protects against the false comfort of the omnivore label. Omnivore is often used to flatten the entire issue into permission. Humans can eat many things, therefore the hierarchy must not matter. But the body's flexibility is not proof of equal suitability. It is proof of adaptive range. Facultative keeps that range visible without pretending the range is nutritionally flat. A person can include some plant foods and still be building the diet on animal foods as the real base. Another may need to keep plant exposure very low because the tradeoffs are not worth it. Another may use carbohydrate more intentionally around heavy training while still relying on protein and fat to anchor daily stability. None of that breaks the model. It expresses the model properly. The body is being fed from its strongest center while allowing the edges to be adjusted according to tolerance and circumstance.

Rigidity usually appears when the person loses sight of what the diet is for. The point is not to collect forbidden foods and safe foods like badges of identity. The point is to create a pattern of eating that keeps the body fed, calm, structurally supported, and metabolically steady. If that can be done with a small amount of well-tolerated fruit, root, or other plant matter without reigniting hunger, digestive noise, or glucose instability, the framework has lost nothing. If those foods repeatedly create friction, then dropping them is not rigidity either. It is simply accurate accounting. The diet should become stricter only where the body keeps showing that stricter works better. It should remain broader where the body handles breadth without real cost. That is what flexibility means when it is tied to physiology rather than to self-indulgence.

So *facultative* does not mean loose, and it does not mean rigid. It means the body has a clear nutritional base and a real adaptive range. The strength of the framework is that it gives the eater a center strong enough to build on without forcing him to confuse discipline with fragility. Protein and fat remain foundational. Animal foods remain primary. Context is allowed to shape the edges. That is not compromise. That is the word doing its job.

Host Tolerance, Environment, Budget, Culture, and Training Demands

A facultative carnivore framework only stays intelligent if it keeps the body in view while also admitting that bodies live somewhere. Host tolerance matters first because the same food does not create the same digestive and metabolic event in every person. One person can handle a small amount of fruit, a modest serving of tuber, or some fermented dairy without appetite distortion, bowel irritation, or glucose volatility. Another cannot. One person can include occasional plant foods and remain calm, regular, and well fed. Another gets bloating, unstable hunger, skin flare, joint irritation, or a quick return of food focus when those same foods rise. This is not a moral difference and not proof that one person is more evolved, balanced, or disciplined. It means the host is part of the equation. Gastric acid output, bile flow, intestinal integrity, microbial activity, prior metabolic damage, autoimmune burden, kidney stone risk, oxalate handling, thyroid state, sleep quality, and nervous system tone all change what a food costs and what it yields. That is why the framework has to stay physiological. The same plant food can be a small harmless addition in one host and a repeated source of friction in another. The body decides that, not the ideology.

Environment matters next because food is never eaten in a vacuum. Climate changes appetite, fluid loss, salt need, and practical food availability. A person working outdoors in heat, sweating heavily, carrying tools, and eating two large meals is not living the same metabolic life as a sedentary office worker grazing through processed convenience foods. Season changes what foods are easy to obtain, what storage is realistic, and what the body may naturally want more or less of. Modern light exposure, sleep disruption, shift work, and stress also belong here because they alter insulin handling, hunger signaling, and recovery. A metabolism living under chronic artificial stress often handles carbohydrate worse, recovers worse, and seeks quicker reward. The right dietary structure in that environment may need to be simpler, denser, and more repetitive than what would work under calmer conditions. Environment is not background scenery. It changes the workload placed on digestion, endocrine control, and fuel use.

Budget matters because biological truth still has to pass through a grocery bill. A strong framework should not collapse the moment premium cuts disappear. The practical center is still animal protein and natural fat, but the sources can vary. Ground beef, eggs, canned fish, bulk dairy where tolerated, cheaper roasts, shanks, organ meats, broth cuts, and occasional liver often outperform a cart full of processed "health" foods even when the latter looks more modern and colorful. Budget pressure often pushes people toward cheap calories because refined starch, sugar, and seed-oil-based products are heavily subsidized and shelf stable. The result is not just economic compromise. It is biological downgrade. The person buys energy because energy is what the system makes cheap. A facultative carnivore approach has to answer that reality by prioritizing nutrient density per dollar, not by pretending everyone is shopping at a boutique butcher. Muscle meat remains the base. Eggs matter. Organ rotation helps. Natural fat matters. The exact expression can be adjusted without surrendering the hierarchy.

Culture matters too, and it matters more usefully when it is treated as meal structure rather than doctrine. Families eat together. Holidays exist. Religious habits exist. Regional cuisines exist. Hospitality exists. A sustainable dietary pattern has to be able to pass through those realities without the person becoming socially brittle or nutritionally confused. This is where the word facultative keeps the framework from becoming childish. If the base of the diet is strong, then an occasional cultural deviation does not rewrite the physiology. If the body tolerates some starch at a family meal, some fruit in season, or some traditional preparation in a social setting without reigniting the old pattern of unstable appetite and daily dependence, the framework has not been betrayed. But the reverse is also true. Culture should not be used as a sentimental excuse to keep eating foods that repeatedly damage digestion, appetite, skin, mood, or metabolic control. Respecting context does not mean surrendering observation. It means knowing the difference between occasional participation and making a harmful pattern foundational again.

Training demands create their own layer because work changes fuel use, tissue turnover, and recovery needs. A sedentary person trying to repair appetite and metabolic stability may function best with very low carbohydrate exposure and a strong protein-and-fat base. A person lifting hard, sprinting, grappling, or doing repeated glycolytic work may tolerate and sometimes benefit from a somewhat wider carbohydrate range without changing the underlying hierarchy of the diet. The key is that training does not erase the need for complete protein, natural fat, and strong micronutrient density. It only changes how much short-range fuel may be useful around that base. Too many people reverse the order. They let training become an excuse to rebuild the diet on starch and quick sugar, then wonder why hunger, crashes, and body composition become harder to control outside the gym. Training should modify the edges, not replace the center. Protein still comes first because tissue repair still comes first. Fat still matters because stable energy, hormone function, and satiety still matter. Carbohydrate, if used, should be serving performance or recovery, not reclaiming control of the whole food pattern.

That is how these variables should be read together. Host tolerance determines what the body can live with cleanly. Environment determines what pressures are acting on the system. Budget determines what form the hierarchy can take in the real world. Culture determines where flexibility has to exist without confusion. Training determines whether some additional fuel flexibility is useful. None of these overturn the central logic. They only shape how tightly or loosely the framework has to be expressed in practice. The foundation remains the same. Foods are judged by biological yield, digestive cost, satiety value, and structural contribution. Context changes the edges. It should not be allowed to erase the center.

Different Levels of Strictness

Different levels of strictness make sense because the body does not always need the same degree of protection in order to stay stable. The mistake is to imagine that a diet is either pure or failed, as though physiology cannot tell the difference between a daily burden and an occasional exposure. It can. A person with severe digestive irritation, unstable appetite, autoimmune flares, skin reactions, migraines, kidney stone history, or obvious carbohydrate volatility often needs a stricter pattern because the body is already showing that small deviations create outsized consequences. Another person with calmer digestion, better metabolic flexibility, and fewer obvious reactivity patterns may do well with a broader range while still keeping animal foods as the unquestioned base. Strictness is therefore not a moral badge. It is a tool for matching the diet to the amount of friction the body can tolerate without losing control of appetite, bowel function, energy, and tissue stability.

At the strictest end, the framework looks like a tight animal-food base with little or no plant matter and almost no exposure to refined carbohydrate, industrial oils, or ultra-processed food. This level is often most useful when the body is noisy enough that clearer signal is needed. The goal here is not asceticism. It is diagnostic and stabilizing. Strip the diet down to the foods that provide the strongest biological yield with the least digestive and endocrine confusion, then watch what happens to hunger, bowel function, sleep, skin, joint irritation, blood sugar stability, and mental quiet around food. A strict phase can show the person what real satiety and metabolic calm feel like once the background noise is removed. For some people that strictness remains the best long-term expression because every attempt to widen the diet simply reopens the same old problems.

A moderate level of strictness keeps the same structure but allows more controlled variation at the edges. Animal foods still form the base. Protein sufficiency still comes first. Natural fats still remain central. But simple plant foods may be added in amounts the body appears to handle well. A modest serving of fruit, a root vegetable, some fermented dairy if tolerated, or an occasional starch used intentionally rather than habitually can fit here without changing the architecture of the diet. What matters is that these foods stay secondary. They do not become the automatic filler on every plate, and they do not return the person to frequent glucose-heavy feeding, unstable appetite, or processed-food logic in cleaner packaging. Moderate strictness works when the body can handle some breadth without losing its center.

A looser level of strictness can still belong inside a facultative carnivore framework if the hierarchy remains intact. This might include more carbohydrate around training, more seasonal variation, more social flexibility, or a wider range of tolerated plant foods in someone who remains metabolically calm and digestively stable with them. But the body still has to earn that looseness. The eater should not confuse tolerance with automatic benefit. A wider pattern is only useful if satiety remains strong, energy remains steady, body composition remains manageable, and the diet does not quietly slide back toward cheap fuel and incomplete completion. Looseness becomes a problem the moment animal foods stop being the nutritional base and start becoming one option among many. Once that happens, the framework has been diluted into ordinary omnivorous drift.

This is why strictness should be judged by results, not by ideology. A stricter pattern is better when it produces more stable appetite, cleaner digestion, better body composition, fewer symptoms, and less food noise. A broader pattern is better when it preserves those outcomes while making life easier, more sustainable, or better matched to training and context. The body is the referee. If widening the diet brings back bloating, cravings, volatility, skin issues, sleep disruption, or the constant need to think about food again, then the looseness was too expensive. If it changes little beyond adding some practical range, then the body likely has room for it. Different levels of strictness are therefore not different religions. They are different distances from the center, and the correct distance is the one the body can hold without slipping back into instability.

How to Keep the Framework While Adjusting the Details

Keeping the framework while adjusting the details begins with knowing what the framework actually is. It is not a list of mandatory foods, a purity contest, or a fixed menu frozen in time. It is a hierarchy. Animal foods remain the nutritional base because they provide the strongest biological yield, the most complete protein, the most usable fats, and the most direct route to structural nourishment. Protein sufficiency stays first. Natural fat stays central. Refined sugar, refined starch, industrial oils, and ultra-processed combinations stay out of the foundation because they destabilize appetite and feed the body poorly relative to the energy they deliver. Those are the fixed pieces. The details are everything that sits around them. Meal frequency. Exact cuts of meat. Amount of dairy. Use of eggs. Inclusion or exclusion of certain plant foods. Carbohydrate level. Organ frequency. Training adjustments. Social flexibility. The framework survives as long as the hierarchy survives.

This matters because most dietary drift happens when people start adjusting details without protecting the order underneath them. A person widens the diet a little, then lets starch become the base of the plate again. Another brings back fruit, then sweet taste begins reopening appetite and snacking. Another adds dairy, then the diet becomes mostly cheese, yogurt products, and convenience food while actual protein density falls. Another decides to be flexible socially and gradually becomes flexible three times a day. The problem is not flexibility itself. The problem is losing the center while claiming the framework is still intact. The way to prevent that is simple. Keep asking the same biological questions. Is the meal still built on substantial animal protein. Is natural fat still doing the work of satiety and slower fuel delivery. Are the additions improving the diet or diluting it. Is appetite still calm. Is digestion still clean. Is energy still stable. Is the person still eating from the body's strengths, or just rebuilding the old pattern in a slightly cleaner costume.

Adjusting details therefore has to be done one variable at a time and read through outcome, not through theory. If a person wants to test fruit, starch, fermented dairy, coffee, spices, or a broader meal schedule, the test is not whether the food fits someone's philosophy. The test is what happens next. Hunger timing changes or it does not. Bloating returns or it does not. Skin worsens or it does not. Cravings rise or they do not. Sleep, body composition, bowel function, mood, and mental quiet around food either remain intact or they begin to slip. This is why gradual adjustment is so much safer than casual drift. The body often gives clear feedback when a detail is helping versus when it is reopening the same old instability. But that feedback is easiest to hear when only one major variable changed at a time.

The framework also holds better when the person distinguishes between a strategic exception and a rebuilt habit. A single social meal is not the same physiological event as restoring a daily base of starch and processed food. A period of higher carbohydrate around intense training is not the same as needing carbohydrate at every meal to feel normal. Seasonal variation is not the same as surrendering the structure. The body can usually handle occasional deviations far better than it can handle repeated foundational errors. That is why details can flex without the framework collapsing, but only if the person keeps the difference clear between occasional context and permanent architecture. The architecture is what the body lives on. The exception is what the body passes through.

So keeping the framework while adjusting the details means protecting the center and negotiating only the edges. Keep the animal-food base. Keep protein sufficiency first. Keep natural fat in place. Keep processed industrial food out of the foundation. Then let the details move only as far as the body can tolerate without losing satiety, digestion, energy stability, and structural nourishment. That is how the diet stays alive without becoming vague. The framework remains fixed where physiology is fixed. The details move where context allows.

Conclusion

The body does not eat categories. It does not eat guidelines, labels, public health campaigns, or food mythology. It eats matter from the outside world and then subjects that matter to a ruthless physical test. Can this be broken down. Can it be absorbed. Can it be turned into structure, stable fuel, and regulated signaling. Or will it create more work than value. That is the question underneath everything in this book. The human organism is not maintained by abstract variety or by the moral reputation of a meal. It is maintained by amino acids that can become tissue, by fats that can become membranes and long-duration fuel, by minerals that can sustain electrical gradients and enzyme activity, and by the endocrine and digestive signals that decide how all of that is handled once food enters the body. When nutrition becomes confusing, it is usually because this physical sequence has been replaced by symbolism. The way back is always the same. Return to the structure. Return to the tissue. Return to what the body is actually built from.

That return changes the standard of judgment immediately. A food is not good because it is natural, colorful, traditional, modern, or widely recommended. A food is good to the degree that it fits the organism processing it. Can the stomach acidify it properly. Can bile and pancreatic enzymes handle it efficiently. Can the small intestine liberate useful nutrients from it in meaningful quantity. Does it create strong satiety because the body actually received something worth keeping. Or does it flood the bloodstream with short-range fuel while leaving the tissues underfed and the appetite system unsatisfied. This is why biological compatibility matters more than food reputation. The body keeps a harder ledger than culture does. It counts what was delivered, what was blocked, what was absorbed, what was stored, what was oxidized, and what had to be cleared afterward. That ledger is where nutritional truth lives.

Protein and fat keep emerging as the core nutritional foundation because they answer the body's central needs more directly than the modern diet usually does. Protein supplies the amino acids required for repair, enzymes, immune function, gut lining turnover, connective tissue, and muscle maintenance. Fat supplies slower fuel, membrane structure, steroid hormone substrate, bile-responsive digestive coherence, and the lipid context required for absorption of fat-soluble vitamins. Together they create meals that the body can interpret clearly. Real satiety rises. Energy becomes less frantic. Feeding stops being a sequence of glucose rescue events and becomes a calmer process of nourishment. This does not mean all other foods are impossible. It means the hierarchy matters. The body needs building material first, stable fuel second, and optional foods only after those first demands are securely met.

Plant foods therefore belong in the diet only to the degree that they help rather than interfere. They are not automatically evil, and they are not automatically foundational. They are conditional foods whose value depends on preparation, dose, host tolerance, metabolic context, and what they displace. Some people will include more. Some will include very little. Some will discover that a small amount of fruit or root fits easily inside a protein-and-fat-centered pattern. Others will discover that even modest plant exposure reopens digestive friction, unstable appetite, skin issues, bowel irritation, or food noise. The important point is that plant foods no longer receive automatic authority. They are judged by yield and cost like everything else. That is a more honest standard and a more humane one, because it lets the body speak instead of forcing the body to obey a reputation.

Feeding the human structure means building the diet from the inside out. Start with what the organism must have. Choose foods that digestion can turn into real nourishment with high yield and low friction. Remove the foods that overfeed energy while underfeeding the body. Let appetite become quieter because the meal is more complete. Let energy become steadier because fuel is arriving in a slower and more durable form. Let food return to its proper role, not entertainment first, not ideology first, not identity first, but biological input first. Once that order is restored, the subject becomes much easier to see. The body was never asking for modern nutrition to be clever. It was asking to be fed according to its design.

Return to First Principles

Return to first principles means stripping nutrition back down to the biological event before culture, marketing, and ideology get the chance to distort it. Food enters the body as outside material. The digestive tract has to break it apart, the intestine has to extract something useful from it, the liver has to sort what was absorbed, the bloodstream has to carry it, and tissues have to either build with it, burn it, store it, or clear what they cannot use. That is the sequence. Every serious nutritional question begins there. Not with whether a food has a good reputation, not with whether it belongs to a fashionable pattern, and not with whether a label can be made to look reassuring. First principles begin with anatomy and chemistry. What is the body made from. What does it need repeatedly. What can digestion actually liberate. What creates friction. What creates yield. What burdens elimination. Once those questions are restored, much of modern nutrition stops looking profound and starts looking evasive.

The body is not maintained by calories in the abstract. It is maintained by amino acids, lipids, minerals, vitamins, water, and controlled signaling. Amino acids are needed because enzymes, transport proteins, immune proteins, connective tissue, gut lining, and muscle all have to be rebuilt continuously. Lipids are needed because membranes, myelin, bile acids, steroid hormones, and long-duration fuel all depend on them. Minerals are needed because electrical gradients, oxygen handling, enzyme systems, and structural integrity depend on them. Vitamins are needed because the machinery that turns food into usable life does not run without cofactors. This is why first principles always pull the discussion away from superficial food talk and back toward tissue economics. The real question is never just what a food contains. The real question is whether the body can turn that food into the materials it is actually built from.

This is also why digestion has to be placed back at the center. A food can test rich in nutrients and still deliver poorly if those nutrients remain bound in the gut, trapped in defended plant structure, diluted by indigestible bulk, or paired with compounds that interfere with absorption. Another food can look simple and outperform it because the stomach can denature it, bile can emulsify it, enzymes can cut it, and the small intestine can absorb it with relatively high efficiency. First principles force the distinction between label content and biological delivery. They also force the distinction between energy and nourishment. A food can provide fast fuel and still fail the body structurally. A meal can fill the stomach and still leave the tissues underfed. Once that becomes visible, the modern obsession with categories starts to weaken. The body is not judging foods by category. It is judging them by what they cost and what they yield.

Return to first principles also means putting hierarchy back into the conversation. Not every edible thing deserves foundational status. The body requires complete protein and useful fats more urgently than it requires dietary diversity for its own sake. It can tolerate a wide range of foods, but tolerance is not the same as optimal fit. A food that supplies dense amino acids, usable fats, fat-soluble nutrients, and strong satiety with relatively low digestive friction belongs in a different rank from a food that requires soaking, fermenting, grinding, fortifying, and careful tolerance management just to become reasonably compatible. First principles do not flatten that difference. They sharpen it. They ask which foods most directly support structure, energy stability, and regulatory order, and which foods are at best conditional additions layered on top of that base.

That is the value of returning to first principles. It clears the subject. Food stops being a moral drama and becomes a biological input again. The body stops being treated like a black box and starts being treated like a living structure with real material needs, real digestive limits, and real metabolic priorities. Once that correction is made, the rest of the framework becomes much easier to hold. Feed the organism what it is made from first. Judge every other food by what it adds, what it displaces, what it costs to process, and what remains after the full event is over. That is where nutritional clarity begins.

The Body Is Built From Amino Acids, Lipids, Minerals, and Regulated Signaling

The body is not built from food groups or dietary ideas. It is built from raw materials that have to be digested, absorbed, transported, and turned into living structure. Amino acids form the protein economy of the organism. They become enzymes, transport proteins, muscle fibers, immune molecules, collagen, receptors, peptide hormones, and much of the repair machinery that keeps tissue from wearing down faster than it can be rebuilt. Lipids form the other half of the architecture. They build membranes, insulate nerves, supply cholesterol for steroid hormone production, provide bile acid substrate, and serve as long-duration fuel when the body is not being driven by constant glucose exposure. Minerals hold the whole system together electrically and chemically. Sodium, potassium, calcium, magnesium, iron, zinc, copper, iodine, selenium, phosphorus. These are not decorative micronutrients riding along at the edge of the story. They maintain gradients, carry oxygen, activate enzymes, stabilize structure, and allow cells to convert food into ATP without losing order. When the body is fed poorly, it is these materials that become thin first, long before the person runs out of calories.

But the organism is not only built from material. It is also built from regulated signaling. That is the part nutrition culture keeps flattening. A meal does not simply add matter to the system. It tells the system what kind of world it is living in. Insulin signals that incoming fuel is here and must be distributed. Glucagon signals that internal reserves should be mobilized. Leptin reports on longer-term energy storage. Ghrelin pushes hunger forward. Cholecystokinin and peptide YY help shut a meal down when meaningful digestion is underway. Thyroid hormone changes the pace of energy turnover. Cortisol changes how urgently fuel has to be made available. These signals do not float above the body as abstract controls. They are the operating instructions that decide what happens to the amino acids, lipids, and minerals once they arrive. Build with this. Burn this. Store this. Release this. Slow down. Speed up. Eat again. Stop eating. The meal is being interpreted at every step.

This is why nutrition cannot be reduced to energy alone. A food can contain calories and still fail the body if it does not deliver enough amino acids for repair, enough lipid material for membranes and hormones, enough minerals for enzyme systems and electrical control, or a meal structure strong enough to produce coherent signaling. The body can be overfed in fuel and underfed in construction at the same time. That is the defining error of the modern diet. It keeps supplying disposable energy while undersupplying the materials and signals that make a human body stable, repairable, and metabolically calm. Once the subject is brought back to this level, the hierarchy becomes harder to ignore. The best foods are the ones that supply these building materials directly and trigger a cleaner regulatory response while doing it. Everything else has to justify itself after that.

Why Biological Compatibility Is the Real Dietary Standard

Biological compatibility is the real dietary standard because the body does not care what a food is supposed to mean. It cares what it has to do with it. A food enters the mouth carrying structure, chemistry, and burden. The stomach has to acidify it or it does not. Bile has to emulsify it or it does not. Enzymes have to cut it into absorbable units or they do not. The intestine has to move those units across a membrane in useful quantity or it does not. The liver has to sort what arrives, tissues have to use it, and the kidneys or bowel have to clear what remains. That full sequence is what makes a food good, neutral, costly, or destabilizing. Reputation is irrelevant at that level. The label can say nutrient-dense, natural, whole grain, plant-based, balanced, or heart healthy. None of that forces the gut to absorb the food well or the tissues to benefit from it. Biological compatibility asks the only question that survives contact with physiology. Does this food fit the organism processing it.

That standard is harder than most nutrition language because it refuses to stop at content. Presence is not delivery. A food can contain calcium, iron, omega-3, protein, antioxidants, or fiber on paper and still yield very little if those compounds remain trapped in the matrix, bound in the lumen, poorly emulsified, badly digested, or paired with chemistry that creates more friction than value. Another food can look plain and deliver far more because its protein is complete, its fats are usable, its minerals are bioavailable, and its digestion runs through the human tract with relatively low resistance. This is why compatibility matters more than virtue. The body is not asking whether a food sounds healthy. It is asking whether it can actually turn that food into tissue, stable fuel, and orderly signaling without paying too much for the privilege.

Biological compatibility also forces food to be judged across organs rather than through one narrow metric. A meal is not only a blood sugar event. It is also a gastric event, a biliary event, a pancreatic event, an intestinal event, a hepatic event, and often a renal event later. A food may look acceptable at the level of calories and still fail at the level of appetite. It may look rich in minerals and still burden the kidney through oxalate handling. It may improve one laboratory marker and still weaken satiety, digestion, or nutrient sufficiency. A compatible food is one that performs well across the sequence, not perfectly in every respect, but well enough that the body is left more supported than burdened when the event is over. That is a much higher bar than simply being edible or socially approved.

This is why protein and natural fat keep rising to the center under this standard. They tend to fit thc human system more directly. Protein supplies amino acids the body repeatedly needs and cannot synthesize in full. Natural fat supports membranes, hormones, bile-responsive digestion, slower fuel delivery, and fat-soluble nutrient absorption. Animal foods often bring these inputs in forms the stomach, intestine, and tissues can use with high yield. Plant foods can still be included, but once compatibility becomes the standard, they lose their automatic authority. They become conditional foods judged by tolerance, preparation, digestive cost, and what they displace. Some may fit. Some may not. Compatibility, not cultural prestige, decides that.

So biological compatibility is the real dietary standard because it restores the missing middle of nutrition. It brings the subject back to anatomy, digestion, absorption, tissue use, and excretion. It stops asking what a food promises and starts asking what the body is actually left with. That is where nutritional truth lives.

Why Protein and Fat Function as the Core Nutritional Foundation

Protein and fat function as the core nutritional foundation because they answer the body's two deepest material questions at once. First, what will the organism be built from. Second, what will it run on without destabilizing itself. Protein answers the structural question because amino acids are the raw material for enzymes, transport proteins, immune molecules, connective tissue, muscle, gut lining turnover, and repair across every organ system. Fat answers the energetic and structural question together because lipids are built into membranes, myelin, bile acids, and steroid hormones while also serving as the body's main long-range fuel. A diet can be high in carbohydrate and still fail both questions if the protein is weak, the fat is thin or industrially distorted, and the meal keeps supplying short-range glucose faster than it supplies the material required to maintain tissue. That is why protein and fat belong at the center. They do the hardest work.

Protein has to sit first because the body cannot improvise around missing amino acids. It cannot turn stored fat into leucine, lysine, methionine, or the other essential amino acids it must obtain from food. If protein is inadequate, the organism starts borrowing from itself. Muscle becomes a source. Repair slows. Enzyme turnover and immune resilience become harder to sustain. The body can tolerate low carbohydrate because it can make glucose where needed through gluconeogenesis. It cannot tolerate low protein indefinitely without structural consequences because the materials for rebuilding have to come from somewhere. This is why a meal built on complete, digestible animal protein changes appetite so powerfully. It does more than provide energy. It tells the body that real substrate for maintenance and repair has arrived in useful quantity.

Fat belongs beside it because a body built only on protein without enough useful fat becomes lean in the wrong way. It may carry amino acids, but it loses part of the digestive timing, membrane support, hormonal substrate, and slower fuel stability that make meals feel complete and metabolism feel calm. Fat changes the shape of the meal. Gastric emptying slows. Bile is recruited. Fat-soluble nutrients become absorbable. Energy enters circulation on a longer timeline. The body stops having to rely so heavily on repeated glucose-heavy feeding just to feel normal. At the cellular level, lipids become membrane architecture. At the endocrine level, cholesterol becomes steroid hormone substrate. At the metabolic level, fatty acids become long-duration fuel. So fat is not there to make food richer in a superficial sense. It is there because the organism is lipid-dependent from the membrane upward.

This is why protein and fat together create a different physiological experience from carbohydrate-centered eating. A carbohydrate-heavy meal can solve immediate fuel need quickly, but it often leaves the deeper nutritional work incomplete if protein and fat are weak. A protein-and-fat meal tends to create stronger satiety because it supplies amino acids the body needs and fuel the body can use over longer intervals. The body reads that as completion. Hunger stays quieter because the meal did more than raise blood sugar. It fed the organism structurally and metabolically at the same time. That does not make carbohydrate useless. It makes carbohydrate secondary. It may have a place, but it is not the foundation because it does not build enough and it does not steady the system enough to carry that role well on its own.

So when protein and fat are called the core nutritional foundation, the claim is not ideological. It is anatomical, digestive, and metabolic. These are the nutrient classes most directly tied to what the body is made from, how it absorbs real nourishment, how it sustains energy between meals, and how it maintains order across tissues over time. Everything else should be judged after those needs are securely met, not before.

Why Plants Remain Context-Dependent Additions Rather Than Automatic Dietary Anchors

Plants remain context-dependent additions because the human body does not meet them as simple nourishment. It meets them as variable chemical packages whose value depends on structure, preparation, dose, host tolerance, and what else is already anchoring the diet. A plant food may contribute carbohydrate, water, flavor, texture, or some useful vitamin and mineral content, but it often arrives with fiber the small intestine cannot fully access, with phytate, oxalate, lectins, tannins, or other compounds that change digestibility and nutrient availability, and with a lower density of complete protein and usable fat than animal foods provide directly. That means the body usually has to negotiate more in order to get less. A food can still be edible under those conditions. It does not become foundational simply because it is edible.

Foundational foods are the foods that answer the body's main recurring demands with the least ambiguity. Complete amino acids, usable fats, fat-soluble nutrient delivery, strong satiety, and relatively direct absorption. Animal foods do that consistently. Plants do it inconsistently. Some roots may provide tolerable carbohydrate in a person who handles them well. Some fruits may be harmless or useful in modest amounts. Some cooked vegetables may add variety without creating major digestive friction. But the key word is some. Their value is conditional. It depends on whether they support the person's appetite, bowel function, energy stability, skin, sleep, and overall metabolic calm, or whether they reopen bloating, cravings, bowel irritation, food focus, mineral interference, or simple displacement of better foods. Once the diet is judged by biological yield, plant foods stop looking like universal necessities and start looking like optional exposures the body either handles well or pays for.

This is why preparation matters so much more with plant foods than with substantial animal foods. A steak needs digestion. A bean often needs soaking, boiling, or pressure cooking before the body can even begin negotiating with it reasonably well. A grain may need milling, fermenting, or long cooking. A leafy plant may still carry a mineral reputation the body never receives because binding chemistry takes the mineral away before absorption. These are not side notes. They are evidence that many plant foods do not present themselves to the human system as direct nourishment. They often need reduction of friction before they become tolerable, and even then the yield may remain modest relative to what a simpler animal food can provide with less negotiation. A food that repeatedly requires disarming before use should not be granted automatic foundational status.

Thinking of plants this way also protects the center of the diet. Once protein and natural fat from animal foods are established first, the body's main structural and energetic needs are already being met. Then a plant food can be judged honestly. Does it add something useful without destabilizing the system. Or does it dilute protein, crowd out fat, increase digestive burden, and pull the meal back toward glucose dependence or bowel irritation. That is the right order. Plants can be included where they fit. They simply do not deserve automatic authority before the body has shown that they help more than they cost. In a facultative carnivore framework, plants remain context-dependent additions because the organism does not need them in order to establish its nutritional base. It only needs them when, and if, they truly improve the result.

Made in the USA
Monee, IL
05 November 2026

67914375R00174